# Creative Psychotherapy

*Creative Psychotherapy* brings together the expertise of leading authors and clinicians from around the world to synthesize what we understand about how the brain develops, the neurological impact of trauma and the development of play. The authors explain how to use this information to plan developmentally appropriate interventions and guide creative counselling across the lifespan.

The book includes a theoretical rationale for various creative media associated with particular stages of neural development and examines how creative approaches can be used with all client groups suffering from trauma. Using case studies and exemplar intervention plans, the book presents ways in which creative activities can be used sequentially to support healing and development in young children, adolescents and adults.

*Creative Psychotherapy* will be of interest to mental health professionals working with children, adolescents and adults, including play and arts therapists, counsellors, family therapists, psychologists, social workers, psychiatrists and teachers. It will also be a valuable resource for clinically oriented postgraduate students, and therapists who work with victims of interpersonal trauma.

**Eileen Prendiville** is the Course Director for the MA in Creative Psychotherapy and Play Therapy at Ireland's Children's Therapy Centre. She is heavily involved in providing play therapy and creative psychotherapy training, both nationally and internationally. She devised 'The Therapeutic Touchstone', an innovative approach for use when working with vulnerable and dependent clients and, with Justine Howard, co-authored *Play Therapy Today: Contemporary practice for individuals, groups and parents*.

**Dr Justine Howard** is an Associate Professor at the College of Human and Health Science at Swansea University. She is a Chartered Psychologist and specialist in developmental and therapeutic play. Her consultancy activity has included the delivery of training courses in play for a wide range of professional groups across children's services. She is internationally recognized as an expert in play and child development, and has published numerous journal articles, book chapters and books in this field.

'This book is a timely and valuable gift to the field of play and expressive arts-based psychotherapy. Neurosequential development is essential knowledge for therapists who work with individuals across the lifespan and specifically to address concerns arising in childhood. Prendiville and Howard have logically sequenced this volume to incorporate neurobiological principles with targeted sensory interventions for lower brain regions and with creative art, narrative and imaginative play interventions to progress neural integration for higher brain systems. A synaptic tree of therapeutic knowledge.'
– **Judi Parson, PhD, RN, APPTA RPT-S: Lecturer in Mental Health – Child Play Therapy, Deakin University, Australia**

'*Creative Psychotherapy* is a fantastic addition to the child therapy literature. This volume offers a wonderfully rich integration of current neurobiological research with various play and expressive therapeutic practices. The worlds of clinical practice and developmental research often exist in parallel. *Creative Psychotherapy* helps bridge these worlds, to the benefit of practitioners, researchers, and most importantly, the children who we try to understand and help.'
– **Henry Kronengold, PhD, Clinical Supervisor, Doctoral Program in Clinical Psychology, City University of New York, USA**

'I enjoyed the book immensely. I felt like I walked right into it and couldn't leave it alone! Some areas I read and re-read several times, then was so intrigued I went to the reference texts to study them. I'm excited to see where this goes!'
– **Joan Wilson, Registered Psychotherapist, Certified Play Therapy Supervisor, Trainer and Supervisor with the Theraplay® Institute, Canada**

# Creative Psychotherapy

Applying the principles of neurobiology to play and expressive arts-based practice

Edited by
Eileen Prendiville and
Justine Howard

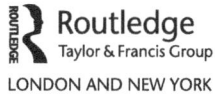
LONDON AND NEW YORK

First published 2017
by Routledge
2 Park Square, Milton Park, Abingdon, Oxon OX14 4RN

and by Routledge
711 Third Avenue, New York, NY 10017

*Routledge is an imprint of the Taylor & Francis Group, an informa business*

© 2017 selection and editorial matter, Eileen Prendiville and Justine Howard; individual chapters, the contributors

The right of the editors to be identified as the authors of the editorial material, and of the authors for their individual chapters, has been asserted in accordance with sections 77 and 78 of the Copyright, Designs and Patents Act 1988.

All rights reserved. No part of this book may be reprinted or reproduced or utilised in any form or by any electronic, mechanical, or other means, now known or hereafter invented, including photocopying and recording, or in any information storage or retrieval system, without permission in writing from the publishers.

Trademark notice: Product or corporate names may be trademarks or registered trademarks, and are used only for identification and explanation without intent to infringe.

*British Library Cataloguing in Publication Data*
A catalogue record for this book is available from the British Library

*Library of Congress Cataloging in Publication Data*
Names: Prendiville, Eileen, 1958–, editor. | Howard, Justine, editor.
Title: Creative psychotherapy: applying the principles of neurobiology to play and expressive arts-based practice/edited by Eileen Prendiville and Justine Howard.
Other titles: Creative psychotherapy (Howard)
Description: Abingdon, Oxon; New York, NY: Routledge, 2017. | Includes bibliographical references.
Identifiers: LCCN 2016005960 | ISBN 9781138900912 (hardback) | ISBN 9781138900929 (pbk.) | ISBN 9781315680507 (ebook)
Subjects: | MESH: Sensory Art Therapies – methods
Classification: LCC RC489.A72 | NLM WM 450 | DDC 616.89/1656 – dc23
LC record available at http://lccn.loc.gov/2016005960

ISBN: 978-1-138-90091-2 (hbk)
ISBN: 978-1-138-90092-9 (pbk)
ISBN: 978-1-315-68050-7 (ebk)

Typeset in Times New Roman
by Florence Production Ltd, Stoodleigh, Devon, UK

Welcome baby Andrew.

Who knew it could get any better? But then there were two – twice as nice. Andrew, there has been much love and laughter, to say nothing about a multitude of hide-and-seek games, with your big sister Emilia. I look forward to the games we will play together – again and again and again. The power of repetition!

I love being a Granny.

Eileen

# Contents

Contributors ix

Introduction 1
*Eileen Prendiville and Justine Howard*

**PART I**
**Applying the principles of neurobiology to play and expressive arts-based practice** 5

1 Neurobiology for psychotherapists 7
   EILEEN PRENDIVILLE

2 Neurobiologically informed psychotherapy 21
   EILEEN PRENDIVILLE AND JUSTINE HOWARD

3 The role of non-directive and directive/focused approaches to play and expressive arts therapy for children, adolescents, and adults 39
   TERRY KOTTMAN, REBECCA DICKINSON AND KRISTIN MEANY-WALEN

4 Counseling skills in action with children, adolescents, and adults 59
   LORRI YASENIK AND KEN GARDNER

**PART II**
**Working with the brainstem and midbrain** 81

5 The role of music and rhythm in the development, integration and repair of the self 83
   EIMIR MCGRATH

6  Being, becoming and healing through movement and touch                   101
   MAGGIE FEARN AND PABLO TROCCOLI

7  Coming alive: finding joy through sensory play                           121
   SIOBHÁN PRENDIVILLE AND MAGGIE FEARN

**PART III**
**Working with the limbic and cortical systems**                            139

8  Art in psychotherapy: the healing power of images                        141
   CLAIRE COLREAVY DONNELLY

9  Sandtray therapy: a neurobiological approach                             157
   DANIEL S. SWEENEY

10 Telling tales: weaving new neural networks                               171
   AIDEEN TAYLOR DE FAOITE, EILEEN PRENDIVILLE
   AND THERESA FRASER

11 A growing brain – a growing imagination                                  185
   KAREN STAGNITTI

   Discussion and conclusion                                                201
   JOAN WILSON

   *Index*                                                                  *209*

# Contributors

## Editors

**Eileen Prendiville** is the Course Director for the MA in Creative Psychotherapy and Play Therapy (Humanistic and Integrative Modality) and the Postgraduate Diploma in Play Therapy, at the Children's Therapy Centre in County Westmeath, Ireland. Eileen was a founder member and National Clinical Director of the Children at Risk in Ireland Foundation, Ireland's specialist treatment service for children and families affected by child sexual abuse. Eileen holds qualifications in Humanistic and Integrative Psychotherapy, Jungian Sandplay Therapy, Biodynamic Psychotherapy and Family Law. She is a psychotherapist, play therapist, supervisor and trainer. Eileen co-edited *Play Therapy Today: Comtemporary practice with individuals, groups, and carers*, published by Routledge, and contributed chapters to this and other books. She was Chairperson of the Irish Association of Humanistic and Integrative Psychotherapy from 2012 to 2014 and is the current Chairperson of the Irish Association for Play Therapy and Psychotherapy. Eileen devised 'The Therapeutic Touchstone', an innovative approach for use when working with vulnerable and dependent clients.

**Justine Howard** (PhD, CPsychol, AFBPsS) is an Associate Professor and Postgraduate Programme Manager in the College of Health and Human Science at Swansea University. She is a Chartered Psychologist and specialist in developmental and therapeutic play. Her consultancy activity has included the delivery of training courses in developmental and therapeutic play for a wide range of professionals across children's services. She has been researching play for more than fifteen years and is internationally recognized as an expert in the field. She has published widely on play and child development and is regularly asked to contribute to national and international conferences and events. Her most recent books include *The Essence of Play* (2013), *Play in Early Childhood* (2010) and *Play Therapy Today* (2014).

## Contributors

**Claire Colreavy Donnelly** (MIACAT, MIAHIP, SIAHIP, MICP) has a BA in Fine Art Installation, Video and Performance Work from NCAD Dublin and an MA in Fine Art from Sheffield Hallam University. She qualified as an art psychotherapist at Sheffield University in 1998. She has worked as a community artist, youth counsellor, art psychotherapist, clinical supervisor and arts therapies trainer. She is an occasional lecturer at CIT, having been a core tutor on the Art Therapy MA in CIT, and now runs the Principles of Art Therapy Course in Dublin, franchised from CIT and hosted by CTC. She has a private practice in Kildare Town and works in an adult psychiatric hospital and an in-patient adolescent unit. She has published articles for *Eisteach*, *Jiacat* and *Inside Out* and has presented at Trinity Healthcare Conferences.

**Rebecca Dickinson** is an Adlerian play therapist who specializes in working with foster and adoptive children. She is a licensed independent social worker and is currently working towards her PhD in Social Work at the University of Iowa.

**Maggie Fearn** (MA DATP, MA Psychotherapy and Play Therapy, BAPT) has been a play practitioner for more than 30 years, gaining an MA in Developmental and Therapeutic Play at Swansea University in 2009, and she has been a Forest School practitioner since 2001. She is a practitioner of Body & Earth experiential anatomy and authentic movement, investigating strategies for supporting developmental movement and sensory awareness during outdoor play. She completed her training as a play therapist and psychotherapist with the Children's Therapy Centre, Ireland, sucessfully achieving her second MA. She facilitates wild play, Forest School and play therapy with children and their families in Wales, and she trains adults in developmental and therapeutic play.

**Theresa Fraser** has worked with children and youth since 1983. Theresa is a certified Canadian play therapy supervisor and has specialized in working with children who have trauma and attachment disruptions for most of her career. She has worked as a professor and is currently a curriculum consultant at Sheridan College in Ontario, Canada. Theresa has written two books, *Billy Had to Move: A foster care story* and *Adopting a Child with a Trauma and Attachment Disruption History*, as well as many articles and book chapters. She is currently working on her PhD in Play Therapy with the University of South Wales.

**Ken Gardner** (MSc, RPsych (CPT-S)) is a registered psychologist with a background in clinical, school and community psychology. As a play therapy supervisor, Ken specializes in assisting children with emotional and/or developmental concerns. Ken is the co-director of the Rocky Mountain Play Therapy Institute and regularly teaches in the area of play therapy, both nationally and internationally. He is the co-author of the *Play Therapy Dimensions Model: A decision-making guide for integrative play therapists*. Ken has also co-authored several chapters on topics such as play therapy supervision, family play techniques and the use of consciousness in play therapy. Ken is a past executive board member of the Canadian Association for Child Psychotherapy and Play Therapy and the Alberta Play Therapy Association.

**Terry Kottman** (PhD, RPT-S, LMHC, NCC) is the 'inventor' of Adlerian play therapy. She is the founder and director of the Encouragement Zone in Cedar Falls, Iowa, a training center for play therapists and other counsellors who work with children and their families. She regularly presents workshops, writes books and plays therapeutically with children at a local elementary school. Terry recently won a Lifetime Achievement Award from the Association for Play Therapy.

**Eimir McGrath** (PhD) is a psychotherapist and play therapist specializing in attachment issues and complex trauma. She has worked in a wide variety of educational and clinical settings and also has extensive experience in working therapeutically with children and adults with disabilities. She is a researcher, lecturer and practitioner in several disciplines, including psychotherapy, play therapy, critical disability studies and dance. Her current research interests are the theoretical application of interpersonal neurobiology to the psychotherapeutic process, the role of creative arts in psychotherapy and the critical analysis of perceptions of disability within society. Her recent publications include chapters contributed to *Disability and Social Theory: New developments and directions* (Palgrave McMillan, 2012), and *Play Therapy Today: Contemporary practice with individuals, groups, and carers* (Routledge, 2014).

**Kristin Meany-Walen** is an Assistant Professor of Counseling at the University of Northern Iowa. She specializes in working with children using play therapy and actively researchers and publishes on the effectiveness and uses of Adlerian play therapy with children. She recently co-authored *Partners in Play: An Adlerian approach to play therapy* (3rd edn) with Terry Kottman.

**Siobhán Prendiville** (BEd, PG Ed, MEd, MA Psychotherapy and Play Therapy) is a teacher and psychotherapist who specializes in the use of play in education and in therapy. She received her play therapy and psychotherapy qualifications at the Children's Therapy Centre in County Westmeath, Ireland. Her main research interests are in the developmental and therapeutic use of puppets, sand and water play, and the pregnant play therapist. She teaches widely in a number of institutions in Ireland: she is involved in training teachers in pilot programmes to influence the teaching methodologies utilized, and in training play therapists. She also maintains a private play therapy practice. Siobhán contributed a chapter on 'Accelerated psychological development' to the second edition (2014) of Dr Charles Schaefer's seminal text, *The Therapeutic Powers of Play: 20 core agents of change*, co-authored with Dr Athena Drewes. She has also contributed a chapter to *Play Therapy Today: Contemporary practice with individuals, groups, and carers* (Routledge, 2014).

**Karen Stagnitti** currently works as Professor, Personal Chair at the School of Health and Social Development at Deakin University, Victoria, Australia. Over the past 30 years and more, she has mainly worked in early childhood intervention programmes in community-based settings as part of a specialist paediatric multidisciplinary team. In 2003, she graduated from LaTrobe University as a Doctor of Philosophy. Her area of research is children's play. Karen has written numerous books and book chapters on play and has had more than eighty national and international papers published. Her norm referenced standardized play assessment, the Child-Initiated Pretend Play Assessment, has been used in several research studies examining: relationships between pretend play, language and social skills; social–emotional understanding and play complexity; play ability in children with autism spectrum disorder; and abilities of children who attend different types of school curriculum. She developed the Learn to Play Therapy programme for children with developmental difficulties who did not have play skills. This programme is now used in several countries.

**Daniel S. Sweeney** (PhD, LMFT, LPC, RPT-S) is a Professor of Clinical Mental Health Counseling and Director of the Northwest Center for Play Therapy Studies at George Fox University in Portland, Oregon. A past president of the Association for Play Therapy, Daniel is an active clinician, international presenter and author/co-author of several books, including: *Play Therapy Interventions with Children's Problems*, *The Handbook of Group Play Therapy*, *Sandtray Therapy: A practical manual*, and *Group Play Therapy: A dynamic approach*. His books have been translated into Chinese, Korean and Russian. Daniel and his wife live in Portland, Oregon, near their four adult children and grandchildren.

**Aideen Taylor de Faoite** is a play therapist and educational psychologist. Having completed the first play therapy course offered in the British Isles, she went on to introduce play therapy to Ireland and set up the Irish Institute for Play Therapy. Over the past 25 years, she has practised as a play therapist and play therapy supervisor. Having trained in a range of theoretical orientations, Aideen continues to contribute to the development of the narrative play therapy model through writing and contributing to various play therapy books.

**Pablo Troccoli** (MAR, RSMT) was educated in Fine Art in Buenos Aires and Boston and began his training in contemporary dance and the study of somatic disciplines applied to movement research, in Berlin. He has professionally performed dance works in multiple collaborations in Germany, Belgium and France. As a somatic practitioner and dance researcher, he holds an IBMT Diploma, the ISMETA accreditation as Somatic Movement Therapist, and a Master of Art by Research degree. He currently resides on a privately owned natural reserve in West Wales, where he is simultaneously extending the boundaries of the dance studio into the landscape, affirming an embodied understanding of human existence and developing his somatic therapeutic skills immersed in a pristine natural environment.

**Joan Wilson** is a registered psychotherapist and certified play therapy supervisor who works from the perspective of attachment and developmental trauma. As well, she brings her training in dyadic developmental psychotherapy and narrative therapy to her work with children, youth and their families. She is a trainer and supervisor with the Theraplay® Institute, travelling around the world to share her knowledge and experience. Joan loves to learn and is excited to be doing this work at a time when the knowledge bases of neuroscience and therapy are being integrated, creating a map for clinical decision-making and planning.

**Lorri Yasenik** (PhD, MSW, RPT-S, CPT-S) is a co-director of the Rocky Mountain Play Therapy Institute in Calgary, Alberta, Canada. Lorri is the co-author of *Play Therapy Dimensions Model: A decision-making model for integrative play therapists* (2012), as well as many book chapters on play therapy supervision and play therapy techniques. Lorri is a certified and registered play therapist supervisor and a founding member of the Alberta Play Therapy Association. She trains nationally and internationally in the areas of play therapy, child psychotherapy, attachment, trauma and high conflict separation and divorce.

# Introduction

*Eileen Prendiville and Justine Howard*

> Play therapy is the only form of therapy that incorporates the core elements of regulation.
> (Bruce D. Perry, APT Conference, 2014)

This book is aimed at therapists who wish to introduce a creative focus into their practice or expand it, so as to work in a more attuned and informed manner with child, adolescent and adult clients. In recent years, it has become widely recognized that professionals can make beneficial use of neurobiological evidence when planning developmentally appropriate and sequential interventions for their clients (Perry, 2006; Perry and Szalavitz, 2006; Perry and Hambrick, 2008; Jennings, 2011; Gil, 2013; Chapman, 2014; Gaskill and Perry, 2014). However, many psychotherapists are searching for clear guidance on how to choose clinically appropriate play- and arts-based interventions to suit the needs of particular clients at various stages of their therapy process. Challenges also exist in terms of timing such interventions within a specific therapy session to ensure that the client is appropriately regulated throughout. An integrated understanding of play (Brown and Vaughan, 2009), the neural system, interpersonal neurobiology and creative therapies (Carey, 2006; Green and Drewes, 2014; Kestly, 2014; Malchiodi, 2014; Malchiodi and Crenshaw, 2014; Badenoch and Kestly, 2015) can inform such decision-making.

The premise of this book is that the planning of sequential creative interventions can be usefully informed by synthesizing what we know about the development of play, the impact of trauma at particular stages and the development of the neural system. Influenced by the neurosequential model of therapeutics (Perry, 2006; Perry and Hambrick, 2008), this book will consider both play therapy and expressive arts interventions that can be used sequentially for healing and brain development. This initially involves movement, music and sensory play and, later, the introduction of art, small world play, organized games, storytelling and dramatic play.

Therapists can make use of bottom–up or top–down approaches (MacKinnon, 2012: 215). Individuals with highly aroused stress response systems require therapeutic interventions that help regulate the lower brain areas. The bottom–up routes rely on somatic and sensory activities and make use of pathways that begin to be developed in utero and are refined through repetitive, rhythmic movement, attuned caregiving and co-regulation, particularly in the early years. Such experiences build and organize neural networks in the brainstem and diencephalon, the least malleable brain regions in later years, and combine to create the embodied experience of safety.

A well-functioning vagal system assists us in remaining calm in situations of safety and where relaxation is desired, becoming appropriately alert in circumstances where increased attention and concentration are beneficial (e.g. in a learning situation), and in responding appropriately in situations of danger. This can be seen in well-modulated levels of arousal and calmness, the outward manifestation of well-functioning accelerator and brake functions associated with the autonomic nervous system.

Although distress interferes with the ability to make use of even well-developed cognitive functions, top–down approaches can be very effective for relatively healthy individuals with a well-organized cortex, who may be struggling to adjust to a new situation or attempting to gain mastery over disturbing emotions or symptoms. Healthy development supports cortical development and promotes strong executive functioning, facilitating advanced capacity to modulate stress responses. Unfortunately, chaotic experiences and developmental trauma compromise cortical development and inhibit the development of neural networks between the neocortex and limbic system – necessary for effective top–down regulation. Children with a poorly organized cortex and a highly reactive stress response are least able to benefit from top–down approaches and will benefit from the safety provided by the use of developmentally appropriate play and creative interventions that allow for the safe processing of implicit, embodied memories.

Clients with a poor capacity to stay regulated are easily triggered into states of hyper- or hypo-arousal when they experience fear, triggers to previous stressors or simply a novel situation that provokes anxiety. The 'window of tolerance' (Siegel, 2012) refers to the zone of optimal autonomic and emotional arousal, within which the system effectively processes internal and external stimuli. A therapeutic aim is to expand the size of this window so that the client can develop the capacity to deal more effectively with stressors, while remaining regulated. This requires development of neural networks between the limbic system and the prefrontal cortex so that the client can pay attention to their here-and-now experiences, tolerate higher-intensity emotions and enhance the capacity of the cortex to calm inappropriate fears by engaging in reality checks – e.g. 'it is not a snake, it is a stick', or 'Mummy will be back to collect me after school finishes'. In this way, the window of tolerance expands.

Play and expressive arts-based therapies facilitate the emergence of unresolved material safely and in symbolic form, thus allowing the social engagement system to remain active and contributing to the development of new neural pathways. The therapeutic relationship and creative therapeutic process engage both right and left brain and support the reworking, and reconsolidation with amended emotional tone, of old memories. In this way, negative world-views shift and are replaced by healthier, positive beliefs and embodied expectations.

## Note

Throughout the book, the names of clients who appear within case studies have been omitted or changed for confidentiality reasons. Some case studies are based on composite case material.

## References

Badenoch, B., and Kestly, T. (2015). Exploring the neuroscience of healing play at every age. In A.L. Stewart and D.A. Crenshaw (eds) *Play Therapy: A comprehensive guide to theory and practice* (pp. 524–38). New York: Guilford Press.

Brown, S., and Vaughan, C. (2009). *Play: How it shapes the brain, opens the imagination, and invigorates the soul*. New York: Avery.

Carey, L. (2006). *Expressive and Creative Arts Methods for Trauma Survivors*. London: Jessica Kingsley.

Chapman, L. (2014). *Neurobiologically Informed Trauma Therapy with Children and Adolescents: Understanding mechanisms of change*. New York: Norton.

Gaskill, R., and Perry, B.D. (2014). The neurobiological power of play: Using the neurosequential model of therapeutics to guide play in the healing process. In C. Malchiodi and D.A. Crenshaw (eds) *Play and Creative Arts Therapy for Attachment Trauma* (pp. 178–94). New York: Guilford Press.

Gil, E. (2013). Integrating a neurosequential approach in the treatment of traumatized children. Interview with C.F. Sori and S. Schnur. *The Family Journal: Counseling & Therapy for Couples & Families*. DOI: 10.1177/1066480713514945.

Green, E., and Drewes, A. (2014). *Integrating Expressive Arts and Play Therapy with Children and Adolescents: A guidebook for mental health practitioners and educators*. Hoboken, NJ: Wiley.

Jennings, S. (2011). *Healthy Attachments and Neuro-Dramatic-Play*. London: Jessica Kingsley.

Kestly, T.A. (2014). *The Interpersonal Neurobiology of Play: Brain-building interventions for emotional well-being*. New York: Norton.

MacKinnon, L. (2012). The neurosequential model of therapeutics: An interview with Bruce Perry. *Australian & New Zealand Journal of Family Therapy*, *33*(3), 210–18.

Malchiodi, C.A. (2014). Neurobiology, creative interventions and childhood trauma. In C. Malchiodi (ed.) *Creative Interventions with Traumatized Children* (2nd edn, pp. 3–23). New York: Guilford Press.

Malchiodi, C.A., and Crenshaw, D.A. (eds) (2014). *Creative Arts and Play Therapy for Attachment Problems*. New York: Guilford Press.

Perry, B.D. (2006). The neurosequential model of therapeutics: Applying principles of neuroscience to clinical work with traumatized and maltreated children. In N.B. Webb (ed.) *Working with Traumatized Youth in Child Welfare* (pp. 27–52). New York: Guilford Press.

Perry, B.D. (2014). Keynote Address to APT Annual Conference, 10 October 2014, Houston, TX.
Perry, B.D., and Hambrick, E.P. (2008). The neurosequential model of therapeutics. *Reclaiming Children & Youth, 17*(3), 38–43.
Perry, B., and Szalavitz, M. (2006). *The Boy Who Was Raised as a Dog.* New York: Basic Books.
Siegel, D. (2012). *The Developing Mind: How relationships and the brain interact to shape who we are* (2nd edn.). New York: Guilford Press.

Part I

# Applying the principles of neurobiology to play and expressive arts-based practice

This part provides an introduction to the ways in which the principles of neurobiology can inform best practice in play and expressive arts-based psychotherapy. The central components of the neurosequential model are introduced, and readers learn how the most effective therapeutic interventions take account of a client's age, developmental stage, experiences of trauma, as well as presenting clinical issues. A case is made for the importance of play and expressive art-based practice across the lifespan for healing and, in particular, for the development and reprogramming of neural networks. A selection of psychotherapeutic approaches are discussed in relation to the level of direction given to the client. An introduction to the evidence base for these different approaches to psychotherapy is provided for clinical work across the lifespan. Finally, before moving on to more specific evidence-based techniques in Parts II and III, the skills associated with creative psychotherapy are considered, and trauma-informed expressive art therapy (Malchiodi, 2014) is presented as one possible framework for integrating the neurosequential model with play and expressive arts-based practice.

Chapter 1

# Neurobiology for psychotherapists

*Eileen Prendiville*

This chapter introduces the reader to neurobiology that is relevant to, and informs, a neurosequential framework and emphasizes the importance of using this to shape psychotherapeutic interventions for young children, adolescents and adults, so that corrective, developmentally appropriate and creative experiences can be identified and offered. Planning appropriate, sequential interventions requires that account is taken of the age of the client, their stage of development, any developmental trauma issues and their clinical presentation. The environment shapes neurobiological development and attachment formation; a creative neurosequential approach to therapy maximizes potential for healing and promotes new neurological development by attending to what we now know about neuroscience, interpersonal neurobiology and the biology of both attachment and arousal.

## The need for playfulness

An understanding of interpersonal neurobiology, trauma and healing suggests that talk therapy alone will not lead to full recovery: there is a need to engage playfully, incorporate some expressive arts into psychotherapy and pay attention to the physiological impact of trauma (e.g. Gantt and Tinnin, 2009; Gaskill and Perry, 2014; Green and Drewes, 2014; Malchiodi, 2014; Malchiodi and Crenshaw, 2014). In discussing the stress response, Perry and Pate (1994) note that talking cannot translate into changes in the midbrain or the brainstem, the very areas that mediate a range of physiological, hyper-reactivity, behavioural impulsivity, hypervigilance, anxiety, emotional lability and sleep problems.

There are different approaches to therapy: top–down models that focus on cognition, and bottom–up models that attend to the central role of physiological elements and the two-way system of brain–body communication. Both left and right brain are involved in healing. The brain's right hemisphere is dominant in the early years of life. It is sensory-based and creative and relies on the somatic, embodied aspects of experience rather than verbal language. It processes social and emotional experiences and is significantly involved in emotional- and self-regulation (Cozolino, 2010; Porges, 2011a: 138–40). The right hemisphere is predominantly activated in the recall of both early and disturbing memories (van der Kolk, 2003: 308), suggesting that right brain activities would be helpful in processing unresolved trauma and modifying embodied, implicit memories, particularly when regulation rather than insight is the therapeutic aim.

## Beginning with safety

The experience of safety in therapy is vital in facilitating the client's engagement and healing. That is why play therapists, for example, concentrate so much on structuring responses in the early stages of therapy. Other possibilities include making a contract, agreeing session times, being predictable in responses, using the therapeutic touchstone story (Prendiville, 2014) and embodying Rogers' core conditions (1957). However, if we agree that feeling safe has both physical and emotional components, then perhaps there may be another dimension to consider in establishing initial safety and facilitating trust building? Given that feeling safe or unsafe is physiological in nature and is directly responsive to the environment, and that feeling unsafe triggers involuntary behaviours that are often problematic, there is a real need for a considered approach to assist clients in becoming regulated so that therapy can take place. Therefore, safety needs to be considered both at the beginning of the therapy process and at the start of each therapy session. Interventions linked to the lower brain regions will be useful in this regard.

## Hierarchical development

The neural system develops from the spinal column in a hierarchical bottom-to-top movement, becoming organized from the more primitive lower (brainstem and midbrain), to more sophisticated higher (limbic system and cortical) regions. Stressful intrauterine experiences and/or early developmental trauma negatively impact both this development and the smooth integration of the interconnected functions of the nervous system. This may result in dysregulation and the individual operating from a baseline alarm state in which the frontal cortex (the thinking brain) and the limbic system (the emotional brain) are shut down. This means that only the lower brain areas are activated, and the individual is severely compromised in terms of:

- establishing a feeling of safety;
- processing incoming information;
- successfully engaging with others;
- recognizing emotional states;
- self-regulating;
- organizing their thinking.

Our capacity to regulate levels of arousal, together with our subsequent baseline state, is heavily influenced by our early experiences and emotional environment. Perry (2006) suggests that levels of state arousal range from calm, alert, alarm or fear to terror, depending on which primary and secondary brain areas are in the driving seat. The range here, linked to the five states listed above, is neocortex/subcortex, subcortex/limbic, limbic/midbrain, midbrain/brainstem and brainstem/autonomic. The individual's capacity to think in these states ranges from abstract in the highest level, down to reflexive in the lowest, with concrete, emotional and reactive in between (p. 32). Our baseline state is activated whenever we experience something new or something that triggers earlier stress. It is clear that people whose baseline state is less than calm, and particularly those whose baseline is alarm, fear or terror, will be unable, not unwilling, to formulate appropriate responses or attend to learning or relationships when in a situation that is experienced by them as stressful or novel. Different people experience the same situation in different ways: whereas one person may be fearful or even terrified, another person in the same situation, even at the same time, may well be calm. Reflecting on the personalized responses of individuals is important: it is not appropriate to expect that a traumatized person will be able to pay attention, learn or heal in the same way as others when their baseline state is aroused by incoming sensory triggers.

Creative approaches to therapy can engage effectively with the client's lower brain areas and positively impact on the modulation of the primary regulatory networks by starting with somatosensory interventions – a bottom–up approach. Suitable activities to calm the nervous system and reinstate a sense of safety, thus making the higher neural networks accessible to relationship, growth and development, include repetitive rhythmic activity such as music and movement, healthy touch and sensorial activities (Jennings, 2011; Gaskill and Perry, 2014; Malchiodi, 2014). Repetitive provision of such experiences builds new, healthy neural networks, promotes synaptic plasticity and modulates lower brain overreact-ivity.

## Motivational circuits in the brain

Panksepp (1998) coined the term 'affective neuroscience' to refer to the study of the neural mechanisms of emotion. He identifies play, particularly physical play, as a primary process in the more primitive parts of the brain. He describes play as a core emotional action system, intimately linked to somatosensory information processing (1998). It integrates the motor, visual, auditory and other sensory regions of the brain, supporting cortical and subcortical organization, promoting brain development, enhancing cognitive abilities and facilitating long-term emotional change. The development of the play system is inhibited by unmet physiological needs and stress.

Panksepp (1998) suggests that all mammals have seven primitive emotional operating systems in the limbic and reptilian areas of the brain. Each primary process affective system is either rewarding or punishing. The rewarding emotional patterns are SEEKING, LUST (activated in adolescence), CARE and PLAY. The punishing systems are RAGE, FEAR and PANIC/GRIEF/SEPARATION DISTRESS.

Whereas the Seeking circuit is generally activated, activation of other circuits is linked to either being in or out of contact with those we trust; in general, it is not possible to maintain satisfactory contact with others when the punishing systems are activated. Adequate physiological regulation is needed to support capacity for relationship. However, a therapeutic relationship can be maintained while processing and engaging with feelings of rage, fear and panic within a pretend play situation. 'Although fight/flight and play behaviours both require mobilization, play turns off defensiveness by maintaining face to face social referencing . . . to signal that the intentionality of the movements is not dangerous or hurtful' (Porges, 2011b: 14). In trauma therapy, the experience of 'just playing' inhibits the generalized activation of the survival system and allows for calmness and interpersonal connection, which facilitate the client in gaining empowerment over difficult emotions, sensations and memories (Panksepp, 1998: 283; Porges, 2011a: 276–7).

## Porges and the polyvagal theory

The nervous system receives and responds to information from both outside and inside the body. The 'sixth sense', that of interoception, is important in sensing internal states and bodily processes. The physiological components of this sense are interoceptors located on the internal organs that detect and transmit messages about sensations arising internally. These sensations may be linked to states of hunger, thirst, pain, tiredness etc.; they may also be the physiological components of emotion. External sensory information is also processed by the nervous system, which must balance the demands of the internal viscera with environmental demands. Sensory processing capacity is very individual, and particular difficulties in detection, modulation, discrimination and integration can exist for clients who have specific conditions, have experienced developmental trauma or have not experienced responsive caregiving.

### *Neuroception*

The capacity to accurately distinguish and process information about current levels of safety or threat directly impacts on our ability to read social cues and regulate our behaviour in the presence of other people. Our nervous system processes incoming information from all our senses and evaluates risk via an unconscious process called neuroception (Porges, 2004): this is more diffuse than perception, relies on neural circuits and assists us in evaluating danger and responding appropriately. Polyvagal theory links social behaviour to the evolution of the autonomic nervous system and provides a model for understanding and treating stress and recognizing the impact of neuroception on emotional well-being, mental health and relationships. Faulty neuroception is linked to faulty reactivity and unnecessary changes in physiology and it results in maladaptive behaviours that are often seen in troubled children and clients within the mental health services.

If the environment is experienced as dangerous, social approaches may trigger a response of aggression or withdrawal – the very opposite of behaviours that would be helpful in the making and maintenance of social bonds.

Porges (2004) uses a traffic light metaphor to explain the three possible visceral states that colour our reactions: green for safety, yellow for danger and red for life threat. Each state is associated with environmental stimuli and induces a response that is personalized to the individual and is directly related to the physiological system active at the time. Such responses will either allow us to remain in contact with others or will cause us to disconnect from social engagement. When our neuroception system is working accurately (evaluating risk and modulating vagal output accordingly), we are able to inhibit our defence systems when we are safe, so that we can engage in social interactions and positive attachments, and we can engage our defences when we are unsafe or in the company of untrustworthy people. When in the presence of a frightened or frightening person, a child's defensive measures may be helpful or ineffective, but they are all that the child can do in the circumstances.

## Bidirectionality

Porges's (2011a) polyvagal theory helps us conceptualize the importance of bidirectionality in the regulation of physiological states and understand how regulation influences our behaviours and social interactions. The processing of information is influenced by both physiological and psychological processes and determines the way we engage in social situations. Emotions have physiological components – they are not just experienced in the brain but throughout the body also. Likewise, physiological experiences impact on our emotions and our behaviour. These simple facts are crucial in understanding the physiological, emotional and involuntary behavioural components and consequences when feelings of safety are compromised, either because of a current threat or a triggered response. When a person is overwhelmed by stress, they often need assistance to regulate their physiology. Understanding the importance of the two-way communication between the viscera and the brain provides us with a host of opportunities to make better use of co-regulation strategies when working with traumatized clients and when working with systems involved in supporting such clients. It also provides a solid rationale for early intervention and education to provide children with opportunities to develop skills in self-regulation. Of crucial importance in psychotherapy is that the experience of safety is a prerequisite for the therapeutic relationship: regulation is the starting point for social engagement.

## Social engagement system

The vagal system plays 'a dynamic role in fostering behavioral and psychological interactions with the environment' and plays a vital role in fostering 'motor and psychological processes associated with appropriate engagement and disengagement with the environment' (Porges, 2011a: 104). Porges (2011a) links the social engagement system, which facilitates connection to others, to the 'smart' ventral vagal parasympathetic system: the myelinated branch of the tenth cranial nerve that originates in the brainstem region. The myelination process takes place during the final 3–4 months *in utero* and the first year (and particularly the first 3 months) of life (Pereyra *et al.*, 1992, cited in Porges, 2007). This myelinated vagal circuit is extremely important in the regulation of both the sympathetic nervous system and the second branch (the old, unmyelinated branch) of the vagus. The smart vagal system, unique to mammals, promotes connection between the heart and the head and can facilitate both self-regulation and co-regulation by transmitting and processing (mainly sensory) cues linked to safety or danger.

The myelinated nerve functions as a vagal brake by adjusting the vagal tone of the heart and regulating the visceral state to facilitate mobilization or achieve calmness by promoting self-soothing behaviours and state regulation and enabling the social engagement system to function (Porges, 2007). 'Functionally, the myelinated vagus is calming us, efficiently processing our cardiovascular and metabolic needs, and actively inhibiting the high states of arousal associated with the sympathetic nervous system' (Porges, 2011a: 6). Achieving and maintaining such a state of calmness is also described as immobilization without fear: the capacity to be calm, comfortable with others and open to safe physical contact and make good interpersonal contact.

## Responding to social cues

An obvious fact, often ignored, is that cues from others impact on our response. Good eye contact, a well-modulated voice, regular pitch and tone and smiling generally elicit positive responses from others. The familiar faces and voices of trusted friends activate a specific part of the temporal lobe area of the cortex and facilitate prosocial behaviours and the inhibition of defensive strategies. However, this is contingent on the person feeling safe. A hyper- or hypo-aroused individual, or one with poorly developed social engagement skills, which may be linked to poor myelination of the ventral vagal circuit (Pereyra *et al.*, 1992, cited in Porges, 2007), may not respond prosocially to such cues from others. This can be confusing and distressing for both people involved. Of significance in the support of clients who do not transmit socially engaging cues (perhaps because they are traumatized, have a poorly developed smart vagal system or have an autism spectrum disorder) is that, although the often negative reaction triggered is totally natural, it is not helpful to respond as if their behaviour was deliberate. A capacity to self-regulate is useful in mediating responses to such clients. Parents are used to considering an infant's needs in relation to hunger, distress and tiredness and responding calmly to these physiological needs; it can be a more difficult task to respond in a co-regulating manner to similar needs in an older child or adult, and even more difficult when the source of the stress is not understood.

## Implicit and explicit memory

There are two types of memory: implicit and explicit. The left hemisphere of the brain is involved in explicit memory that is rational and conscious, has associated language and can be used to describe thoughts and feelings and give narrative to past experiences. Explicit memory is associated with the hippocampus and is active from approximately 3 years of age. Implicit memory is based in the right brain and is linked to early experiences, trauma memories and learning through experience on a sensory and somatic level. It is associated with the amygdala and is active from birth. Early implicit memories are rooted in the limbic region and provide the template for our future expectations and world-view. Without language, embodied, implicit memory relies on sensory and emotional elements and is experienced as current. Implicit memory is particularly relevant for therapy work with traumatized clients, because trauma memories are stored as implicit rather than explicit memories.

## The brain and the nervous system

It is outside the scope of this chapter to present detailed anatomical and physiological information, or to address in detail the vast information that is now available to us in relation to the neurological impacts of abuse, neglect or emotionally responsive parenting (e.g. van der Kolk, 2003; Perry, 2006; Sunderland, 2006; Fraser, 2014; Gerhardt, 2014). The purpose here is to provide a basic level of understanding that will ensure foundations are in place to embed the more complex interpersonal neurobiological concepts that are described and discussed at various stages throughout this text.

### *The triune brain*

MacLean first proposed his engaging theory of the triune brain in the 1960s. This is an evolutionary model that hypothesizes that the human brain consists of three distinct groups of interconnected structures, the reptilian brain, the mammalian (emotional) brain and the rational brain, sequentially added to the forebrain in the course of evolution (MacLean, 1990). Each set of increasingly complex structures equips us for more adaptive social behaviours and increases our capacity for self-regulation and empathy when activated in a coordinated fashion. Sunderland (2006: 16–19) makes the theory of the triune brain very accessible. She presents the reptilian brain as the ancient core, surrounded by the mammalian brain and encased by the rational brain. She clearly and simply links the least complex to 'primitive impulses of defence and attack', highlights the middle layer's involvement in emotional life and social behaviour and describes the most evolved, the neocortex, as providing potential for 'highly sophisticated powers of reasoning' and enjoying 'the highest level of social intelligence with the deepest level of compassion and concern'.

- The 'reptilian brain' (brainstem and cerebellum) coordinates basic regulatory functions, reflexes, level of arousal, cardiovascular functions (brainstem), and motor, emotional and cognitive functions (cerebellum).
- The 'mammalian brain' (limbic system or emotional brain) is the source of urges, needs and feelings.
- The rational brain (neocortex) is the higher part of the brain where thinking, planning and problem solving occur. It also provides for self-awareness, imagination and creativity, and empathy.

*Functional divisions within the brain*

Perry (2001) describes the brain as having four interconnected functional divisions – the brainstem, the diencephalon, the limbic system and the cerebral cortex. It is important to note that some of these divisions are not anatomical: for example, the limbic system is grouped according to function, rather than location. The least complex area in terms of structure, cellular organization and function, the brainstem develops first and is followed sequentially by the more complex regions. Physiological functions such as breathing, body temperature, heart rate and blood pressure are regulated by the brainstem (hindbrain). The midbrain is involved in regulating motor activity, sleep and appetite. The limbic system is involved in our levels of emotional reactivity, relationships, attachments and sexual behaviour. More complex functions, such as abstract thinking, decision-making and language, are mediated by the neocortex. Brain development is linked to environment, and the degree of order achieved reflects the degree of regularity and normality of experiences. Irregular, extreme neural activity associated with neglect or trauma disrupts development and compromises future functioning. Later chapters in this text will provide guidance in matching the nature and type of therapeutic intervention offered to client's needs in relation to the brain region(s) and associated functions impacted by their life experiences and exposure to stress.

*The nervous system in a nutshell*

The nervous system has two parts: the central nervous system and the peripheral nervous system. It is this combined system, rather than the brain, that 'controls' the person.

The central nervous system is comprised of the brain and the spinal cord:

- The spinal cord transmits neural messages between the brain and the rest of the body.
- The brain:
    - has two hemispheres connected by nerve fibres – the corpus callosum;
    - is a very complex organ with many interconnected areas;
    - comprises three main parts: the forebrain, midbrain and hindbrain.

The peripheral nervous system also has two parts that work in a coordinated manner – the somatic nervous system and the automatic nervous system:

- The somatic nervous system controls voluntary movement and reflex actions. It sends sensory messages to the central nervous system and motor commands to the muscles, controlling external movement through space.
- The automatic nervous system regulates our physiological processes and provides a communication channel between the viscera (internal organs – 'gut brain') and the brain (skull brain). It is involved in helping us to rest and relax or mobilize; it supports health, growth and restoration in times of calmness and activates our defensive systems in times of stress. This balance is facilitated by the coordinated and complementary functions of the enteric, sympathetic and parasympathetic nervous systems, which are constantly assessing safety levels and responding sequentially to levels of safety/danger detected.
  - The ventral vagal parasympathetic is the first response and actively promotes social engagement in situations of safety. It has a calming function: the primitive defensive systems are inhibited, and engagement in social communication and play is facilitated. This state is linked to optimal levels of arousal.
  - When a person neuroceives the environment as dangerous, the sympathetic system activates the fight or flight response (hyperarousal).
  - In a situation experienced by our neural circuitry as life threatening, the peripheral nervous system is activated and leads to a freeze response of dissociation, shutdown or collapse (hypoarousal).

Thus, the sympathetic system is linked to alertness, mobilization and responding to danger with fight or flight responses, whereas the parasympathetic system can be linked to either immobilization without fear (rest and relaxation) and social connection (in situations of safety) or immobilization with fear (in situations of life threat).

### The stress response: Fight – flight – freeze

Stress responses cause physiological changes (e.g. raising or lowering) in blood pressure, heart rate, temperature, breathing, digestion, metabolism, muscle tone, pain threshold and hormonal and chemical balance. Our bodies are equipped to respond adaptively to danger by either fighting, fleeing or freezing. None of these is intrinsically better or worse than the others. What is significant is the situation itself, the options available to the person and their developmental status. Prior experiences may also be relevant. An adaptive response commonly includes elements of hyperarousal (mobilization for defence) and elements of hypoarousal and dissociation (freeze and surrender) as the dangerous event progresses. Fighting and fleeing (hyperarousal) are action-oriented (sympathetic nervous system) responses that focus attention on the critical components in the external world and options to engage with it defensively. Freezing (hypoarousal) has an inward focus, and attention is drawn to the internal world as a way of reducing awareness of (avoiding) the situation in which one finds oneself (parasympathetic nervous system). Young children have less capacity to fight or flee than adolescents or adults, and therefore compliance and dissociation are common components of the response to childhood trauma. Fighting or fleeing is not possible if you are immobilized or otherwise incapable of escaping an intolerable situation characterized by pain, terror and helplessness.

Common to all stress responses is the cognitive impairment element, as oxygen is diverted from the cortex. This impairment may reduce or eliminate the capacity to accurately evaluate the actual level of danger. Bypassing of the cortical system facilitates the limbic appraisal system to make quick decisions in relation to possible danger. When the amygdala is activated, it emits emotional and hormonal signals to initiate the stress response, which involves the hypothalamic–pituitary–adrenal axis in a host of psychological and physiological fear-based responses: the release of corticotrophin-releasing factor by the hypothalamus and adrenocorticotropic hormone by the pituitary gland, and the secretion of stress hormones (cortisol, adrenaline and noradrenaline) by the adrenal gland.

Ideally, when danger recedes, the state of alarm gradually eases, and a state of calm is restored. This involves the body regaining its normal physiological state, including modifications to heart rate, breathing, blood pressure and digestion, plus the reactivation of the higher areas of the brain (rather than the brainstem and diencephalic stress-mediating neural systems retaining control), so that expressive and receptive language becomes more accessible and thinking is clearer. The person (child, adolescent or adult) regains the capacity to focus appropriately on both internal and external stimuli. The stress response hormones (e.g. cortisol and adrenaline) are deactivated, and the chemical balance in the body will be restored to normal. The time it takes for this to happen is influenced by the resilience of the person, the nature of the support that is available to them and the capacity to re-engage the social engagement system. When the threat is perceived to have receded, the person is now left with a memory of the event that needs to be processed so that a sequential narrative can be given to the experience and they can gain mastery over the extreme emotions evoked and regain a sense of empowerment and control.

## Difficulties with arousal levels

Perry (2001) cautions that the neural system mediating the stress response is disrupted by prolonged activation. Those who experience persistent states of hyperarousal have a compromised ability to evaluate stimuli accurately in terms of the threat they comprise, and their orbitofrontal cortex is unlikely to be fully available for stimulus discrimination, learning and problem solving (van der Kolk, 2003: 307).

Significant problems can be evident when the fight, flight or freeze response is evoked by an 'innocuous stimulus' (van der Kolk, 2003: 305) that is misinterpreted as dangerous in response to trauma-related triggers, or when it becomes a persistent state, rather than being adaptive to a current threatening situation. When this occurs, the arousal state is governed by the more primitive parts of the brain, rather than being responsive to the here and now. Unfortunately, this can lead to further difficulties, as the person's level of arousal makes it impossible for them to regulate their responses, and they exhibit behaviours that are likely to be determined by others as defiant, aggressive or inattentive, rather than an involuntary reaction that would more helpfully be addressed by the availability of regulatory assistance. Instead, we can see a spiral, as angry responses trigger even more primitive reactions while the person attempts to adapt to the situation as they experience it. Stress-related physiological states reduce each individual's capacity to connect with higher, more rational responses, and bad situations quickly deteriorate unless help with regulation is available or utilized.

## Memory storage and the brain

The storage of memories is also associated with the various brain regions discussed earlier. Aspects of memory are stored in the regions associated with their specific functions. Therefore, the cortex is associated with cognitive memory, the limbic system is associated with emotional memory, the cerebellum and midbrain are associated with the motor-vestibular memory (similar to procedural, in that this is the body's way of unconsciously remembering how to repeat regularly occurring actions), and the brainstem is associated with the level of arousal. The right hemisphere is associated with nonverbal and sensory images and implicit memories, and the left is associated with language, linear thought and explicit memories. The emotional and physiological features associated with traumatic events can be triggered by sensory reminders and evoke body memories, physiological reactions and the neuroception of safety, danger or life threat associated with states of hyperarousal or hypoarousal.

One final element to consider at this point is that the nature and location of storage of memories in the brain, and their impact on the individual's development and subsequent functioning, will be influenced by the nature and timing of the event and the area of the brain that is most involved in growth and development at that time. The 'hot zone' (Perry, 2001) that is most rapidly organizing is most influenced by current experiences. Neurons are 'born' while the foetus is still in the womb but, in order to continue to survive after birth, they have to migrate to the appropriate location, mature and become organized, through active use and in response to chemical signals, into functional networks and systems. How these systems connect with others and become organized is impacted by the nature of regularly co-occuring events, the level of activation achieved and the nature of the activation or disruption.

The neuroarcheological perspective suggests that the *specific* dysfunction will depend upon the timing of the insult (e.g., was the insult in utero during the development of the brainstem or at age two during the active development of the cortex), the nature of the insult (e.g., is there a lack of sensory stimulation from neglect or an abnormal persisting activation of the stress response from trauma?), the pattern of the insult (i.e., is this a discrete single event, a chronic experience with a chaotic pattern or an episodic event with a regular pattern?).

(Perry, 2001: 21; emphasis in original)

As the brain develops sequentially, and each area develops over a prolonged period, adverse events may impact on more than one region. Experiences impact most intensely on the system as it develops, literally shaping its development. The brainstem reaches maturity in infancy, the midbrain during childhood. The limbic system is not mature until adolescence, and the cortex continues to develop even in adulthood (Perry, 2001). Each level of development rests and builds on what has been already acquired: it is clear that the most complex functions associated with higher, later-developing areas of the brain (limbic system, subcortex and neocortex) may well be compromised even if the adverse events occurred *in utero* and/or in the early months of life, when the neural system was at its most vulnerable. Memories of these events will likewise be stored in lower brain regions and will be revealed in difficulties associated with regulation, rhythm and sensory processing. The somatic elements of trauma need to be addressed just as much as, and with more immediacy than, the emotional impacts.

## Conclusion

This chapter has laid out some of the main theories and concepts that a neurobiologically informed psychotherapist would rely on in planning and conceptualizing their practice through a neurosequential lens. It is recommended that the psychotherapist have some knowledge of hierarchical development, levels of arousal, primary emotional systems, the brain and nervous system, the stress response and polyvagal theory. In the next chapter, we will consider how these theories may impact on our clinical practice.

## Key points

- The neural system develops in a hierarchical fashion, from lower brain regions up to the neocortex.
- The environment shapes neurodevelopment and attachment formation; the timing of specific experiences determines the impact and the regions involved.
- When fight, flight or freeze responses are activated (either in response to a current threat or as a persistent fear state), our social engagement system is inhibited, and our cortex is 'offline'.
- Play is a core emotional action system that supports integration and neural organization.

## References

Cozolino, L. (2010). *The Neuroscience of Psychotherapy: Healing the social brain* (2nd edn). New York: Norton.
Fraser, T. (2014). How neuroscience can inform play therapy practice with parents and children. In E. Prendiville and J. Howard (eds) *Play Therapy Today: Contemporary practice with individuals, groups, and carers* (pp. 179–98). London: Routledge.
Gantt, L., and Tinnin, L.W. (2009). Support for a neurobiological view of trauma with implications for art therapy. *Arts in Psychotherapy, 36*, 148–53.
Gaskill, R., and Perry, B.D. (2014). The neurobiological power of play: Using the neurosequential model of therapeutics to guide play in the healing process. In C. Malchiodi and D.A. Crenshaw (eds) *Play and Creative Arts Therapy for Attachment Trauma* (pp. 178–94). New York: Guilford Press.
Gerhardt, S. (2014). *Why Love Matters: How affection shapes a baby's brain* (2nd edn). Hove, UK: Routledge.
Green, E., and Drewes, A. (2014). *Integrating Expressive Arts and Play Therapy With Children and Adolescents: A guidebook for mental health practitioners and educators*. Hoboken, NJ: Wiley.
Jennings, S. (2011). *Healthy Attachments and Neuro-Dramatic-Play*. London: Jessica Kingsley.
MacLean, P.D. (1990). *The Triune Brain in Evolution: Role in paleocerebral functions*. New York: Plenum Press.
Malchiodi, C.A. (2014). Neurobiology, creative interventions and childhood trauma. In C. Malchiodi (ed.) *Creative Interventions with Traumatized Children* (2nd edn, pp. 3–23). New York: Guilford Press.
Malchiodi, C.A., and Crenshaw, D.A. (eds) (2014). *Creative Arts and Play Therapy for Attachment Problems*. New York: Guilford Press.
Panksepp, J. (1998). *Affective Neuroscience: The foundations of human and animal emotions*. New York: Oxford University Press.
Pereyra, P.M., Zhang, W., Schmidt, M., and Becker, L.E. (1992). Development of myelinated and unmyelinated fibers of human vagus nerve during the first year of life. *Journal of Neurological Sciences, 110*, 107–13.
Perry, B.D. (2001). The neuroarcheology of childhood maltreatment: The neurodevelopmental costs of adverse childhood events. In K. Franey, B. Geffner, and R. Falconer (eds) *The Cost of Child Maltreatment: Who pays? We all do* (pp. 15–37). San Diego, CA: Family Violence and Sexual Assault Institute.
Perry, B.D. (2006). The neurosequential model of therapeutics: Applying principles of neuroscience to clinical work with traumatized and maltreated children. In N.B. Webb (ed.) *Working with Traumatized Youth in Child Welfare* (pp. 27–52). New York: Guilford Press.
Perry, B.D., and Pate, J.E. (1994). Neurodevelopment and the psychobiological roots of post-traumatic stress disorder. In L. Koziol and C. Stout (eds) *The Neuropsychology of Mental Disorders: A practical guide* (pp. 129–46). Springfield, IL: Charles C. Thomas.
Porges, S.W. (2004). Neuroception: A subconscious system for detecting threats and safety. *Zero to Three, May*, 19–24.
Porges, S.W. (2007). The polyvagal perspective. *Biological Psychology, 74*(2), 116–43. Available at: www.ncbi.nlm.nih.gov/pmc/articles/PMC1868418/ (accessed 4 November 2105).

Porges, S.W. (2011a). *The Polyvagal Theory: Neurophysiological foundations of emotions, attachment, communication, self regulation.* New York: Norton.
Porges, S.W. (2011b). 'Somatic perspectives' series: Interview with Serge Prengel. USABP and EABP. Available at: www.SomaticPerspectives.com (accessed 16 May 2016).
Prendiville, E. (2014). The therapeutic touchstone. In E. Prendiville and J. Howard (eds) *Play Therapy Today: Contemporary practice for individuals, groups, and parents* (pp. 7–28). London: Routledge.
Rogers, C. (1957). The necessary and sufficient conditions of therapeutic personality change. *Journal of Consulting Psychology, 21,* 95–103.
Sunderland, M. (2006). *The Science of Parenting.* London: Dorling Kindersley.
van der Kolk, B.A. (2003). The neurobiology of childhood trauma and abuse. *Child & Adolescent Psychiatric Clinics, 12,* 293–317.

Chapter 2

# Neurobiologically informed psychotherapy

*Eileen Prendiville and Justine Howard*

Psychotherapists working with play and expressive arts-based approaches have long recognized the power of the creative, and many psychotherapists and play therapists are firmly committed to providing developmentally appropriate practice for their young clients.

> In the midst of play, neurotransmitters move towards balance, belly brains relax, heart brains learn something wonderful about relationships, autonomic nervous systems find easy access to the branch that allows us to connect with one another, and old memories of trauma and loss can surface and be reworked.
>
> (Badenoch and Kestly, 2015: 525)

In this chapter, we consider ways in which neurobiological theories and concepts can inform psychotherapy practice with children, adolescents and adults. Relatively recent discoveries in the field of neuroscience provide a new lens through which we can view clinical practice and understand the change process more deeply. For some, this highlights a need for a radical change in practice; for others, the new learning confirms what was known before, and so it prompts less dramatic changes but provides a welcome framework that facilitates new understanding of existing practices. There can be few creative therapists who are not delighted to have a new language to conceptualize and communicate more clearly what they do and why it works from a neurobiological perspective.

Neurobiologically informed psychotherapists take a neuroscientific perspective and are mindful of the biology of attachment and arousal. Such knowledge is used to inform clinical decision-making. We see the benefits of assisting clients to become regulated at the beginning of each therapy session and remain regulated during sessions and of helping clients expand their capacity to remain regulated in novel and/or adverse circumstances. In this chapter, early, proactive engagement with at-risk children and families is advocated. The need to work with and educate family members in regard to the rationale for the treatment modality chosen and the ways in which recovery can be supported is highlighted.

## The 3 Rs and the Embodiment–Projection–Role paradigm

At a training event in the mid 1990s, Anne Bannister, who pioneered the Child Sexual Abuse Consultancy for the National Society for the Prevention of Cruelty to Children in the United Kingdom, talked about the 3 Rs in the therapy process. These 3 Rs are reassurance, re-enactment and rehearsal. Anne made a point that every (play) therapy session will contain all these stages. Not only that, every therapy process has these stages, and she suggested that, in the early stages (of the therapy session and of the therapy process), the main element will be reassurance; in the middle phase, it will be re-enactment; and, in the closing stages, it will be rehearsal. Personal professional experiences have found this to be true: these 3 Rs give a clear way of conceptualizing the individual client's process. Let us take a moment to explore the three stages as they make sense in regard to child clients. Reassurance is not about the therapist reassuring the child; it is about the child becoming reassured that this is a safe place, that the therapist is a safe person, and that it is safe to be in this relationship. In the early stages of therapy, the bulk of the session may be linked to this, with only momentary engagement in the other two Rs. Re-enactment is the stage in which the core work in therapy takes place, where the child engages with whatever is unresolved for them, whatever is interrupting and/or impeding their development, their relationships, their happiness. Again, this is not necessarily therapist-led; once a child feels safe, and we provide an appropriate play environment, they will engage in play that has specific personal relevance and open a window into their world for us. In fact, brief interludes of distress-related play may randomly appear even in the early stages and can be the short re-enactment section of even the first and second sessions. Rehearsal is the stage of practising for the future. In the early days, it is the closing phase of the session, as the child prepares to return to the real world outside the therapy room and the different expectations that may be placed on them in that environment. In the later stages, it is where the child practises for transferring the new skills and a freer, healthier, more mature way of being, learned in therapy, to the outside world. Children commonly engage in role-play of real-life situations during this phase.

Another concept presented by Anne Bannister in that training was Sue Jennings' Developmental Playtherapy method (Jennings, 1999) based on her Embodiment–Projection–Role (EPR) paradigm that uniquely charts dramatic development in the first 7 years of life. This approach emphasizes the importance of providing embodiment (movement- and sensory-based) activities in all therapeutic and developmental interventions prior to engaging in any play outside the body (e.g. using small world materials or role-play). The body is recognized as the primary means of learning, and physical play is presented as a crucial means of working with trust issues, establishing a healthy brain–body connection and developing a body-self. The EPR framework is ideally suited for application in planning therapeutic and creative groupwork (Jennings, 2014). Of note in this approach is the recognition afforded to the therapeutic benefits of early play, play that involves all senses, including proprioception and the vestibular sense. Practitioners frequently encounter a misperception that therapeutic play is mainly based on imaginative play or on play in which the child engages with toys. The importance of pre-symbolic and physical play cannot be overemphasized, and such play is highly effective in helping clients to regulate, overcome stress and accept contact. Exploratory, sensory, rhythmic, embodiment and messy play are all crucial in establishing a sense of trust, which is critical to the psychotherapy and play therapy process. In recent years, we have begun to think about neurobiological influences on the healing process and we are reminded again of the sequential core of both EPR and the 3 Rs and how both of these have been practitioner responses to challenges presented by the neurological impact of trauma on children. Talking about traumatized children, van der Kolk (2003) states:

> The task of therapy is to help these children develop a sense of physical mastery and awareness of who they are and what has happened to them to learn to observe what is happening in the present time and physically respond to current demands instead of recreating the traumatic past behaviourally, emotionally, and biologically.
>
> (p. 311)

## A neurosequential approach to psychotherapy

Neurosequential interventions (Perry, 2006; Perry and Hambrick, 2008; MacKinnon, 2012) are designed to replicate the normal stages of development, beginning with approaches that target the lowest, most primitive parts of the brain. Play is the ideal medium for child therapy (e.g. Jennings, 1999, 2011; Bratton *et al.*, 2005; Gil, 2006, 2010; Brown and Vaughan, 2009; Schaefer and Drewes, 2014; Badenoch and Kestly, 2015), and creative therapies (e.g. Carey, 2006; Gaskill and Perry, 2014; Green and Drewes, 2014; Malchiodi, 2014; Malchiodi and Crenshaw, 2014) have application throughout the lifespan. An individual treatment plan will seek to match the therapeutic activities to the physiological needs, developmental stage and interests of the client, while taking account of the neurobiology of trauma. Perry (2006) has identified six principles of neurodevelopment that have significant implications for clinical practice, as follows:

1 The brain is organized in a hierarchical fashion, such that all incoming sensory input first enters the lower parts of the brain.
2 Neurons and neural systems are designed to change in a 'use-dependent' fashion.
3 The brain develops in a sequential fashion.
4 The brain develops most rapidly early in life.
5 Neural systems can be changed, but some systems are easier to change than others.
6 The human brain was designed for more primitive times and is slowly evolving.

Table 2.1 Sequential neurodevelopment and therapeutic activity

| Age of most active growth | 'Sensitive' brain area | Critical functions being organized | Primary developmental goal | Organizing experiences (examples) | Therapeutic and enrichment activities (samples) |
|---|---|---|---|---|---|
| 0–9 months | Brainstem | Regulation of arousal, sleep and fear states | State regulation | Rhythmic and patterned sensory input (auditory, tactile, motor) | Massage |
| | | | Primary attachment | Attuned, responsive caregiving | Rhythm (e.g. drumming) |
| | | | Flexible stress response | Reiki touch | |
| | | | Resilience | | EMDR |
| 6 mnths–2 years | Diencephalon | Integration of multiple sensory inputs | Sensory integration | More complex rhythmic movement | Music and movement |
| | | Fine motor control | Motor control | Simple narrative | Reiki touch |
| | | | Relational flexibility | Emotional and physical warmth | Therapeutic massage |
| | | | Attunement | | Equine or canine interactions |
| 1–4 years | Limbic | Emotional states | Emotional regulation | Complex movement | Play and play therapies |
| | | Social language; interpretation of | Empathy | Narrative | Performing and creative arts |

| | | | | and therapies |
|---|---|---|---|---|
| | | | | Parallel play |
| | | nonverbal information | | |
| | | Affiliation | Social experiences | |
| | | Tolerance | | |
| 3–6 years | Cortex | Abstract cognitive functions | Abstract reasoning | Complex conversation | Storytelling |
| | | Socio-emotional integration | Creativity | Social interactions | Drama |
| | | | Respect | Exploratory play | Exposure to performing arts |
| | | | Moral and spiritual foundations | Solitude, satiety, security | Formal education |
| | | | | | Traditional insight-oriented or cognitive-behavioural interventions |

Note: This table outlines the sequential development of the brain, along with examples of appropriately matched experiences that help organize and influence the respective parts of the brain that are most actively developing at various stages. For maltreated children, developmental 'age' rarely matches chronological age; therefore, the sequential provision of therapeutic experiences should be matched to developmental stage and not chronological age

Source: Perry, 2006. © Guilford Press. Reprinted with permission of Guilford Press

A neurosequential approach to therapy takes account of sequential neurodevelopment, the need to begin with the least complex brain area and move sequentially through the more complex regions (i.e. brainstem first, then midbrain, then limbic, then cortex), the functions associated with each region (i.e. regulation of arousal, sleep and fear states, somatosensory integration, emotional regulation, concrete and abstract thought) and the types of intervention that best address each area of dysfunction (massage, rhythm, movement, sensation, animal-assisted therapy, play, art, drama, storytelling etc.). An awareness of the brain areas under development at various stages and the related goals of development and associated organizing experiences will inform the choice of therapeutic and enrichment interventions (see Table 2.1, reprinted from Perry, 2006: 41).

Effective therapy will address the developing (or poorly developed) brain region in the mode that is best suited to it. For example, a child experiencing significant difficulties in the brainstem region may best be served initially with embodiment activities and rhythmic, sensory and tactile play approaches. Moving and being moved in space will aid regulation, as will activities that focus on the body, breathing, safe massage and healthy touch.

Some activities address a number of brain regions simultaneously. A child may struggle with hyperarousal but also be capable of cognitive learning. Linking psycho-educational components with physical activity can be beneficial. An expanding ball (e.g. Hoberman's sphere) is a great tool for helping children focus on their breathing: they expand the ball while breathing in slowly and collapse it on the out breath. In practising this style of breathing, they experientially learn its relaxing properties. The ball also serves as a visual aid in learning how the fast breathing that occurs when someone is upset does not expand the lungs, and that they can slow down their breathing when they need help in calming down.

Other clients experience a persistent fear state, and the brainstem is constantly dysregulated. Initial interventions chosen for such clients must address the level of arousal, or else there is little chance of success and significant risk of further traumatization.

> The key to therapeutic intervention is to remember that the stress response systems originate in the brainstem and diencephalon. As long as these systems are poorly regulated and dysfunctional they will disrupt and dysregulate the higher parts of the brain. All the best cognitive-behavioural, insight-oriented, or even affect-based interventions will fail if the brainstem is poorly regulated.
>
> (Perry, 2006: 38–9)

Any intervention that provides patterned, rhythmical, repeated stimulation of the brainstem will contribute to building new neural networks and assist in regulation. These activities can include music, drumming, movement, EMDR and rhythmical touch. There is a strong sensory element to highly charged memories;

the use of active methods in therapy will build bridges between the right and left hemispheres and implicit and explicit memories.

Perry promotes 6 Rs in the planning and implementation of therapeutic interventions:

1 Relational: The first priority is to establish safety, including state regulation, so that connection is possible.
2 Relevant: Intervention should be matched to the developmental needs of the client.
3 Repetitive: Activating neural networks in a repetitive way instigates change.
4 Rewarding: Activities should be enjoyable; avoiding trauma triggers will increase pleasure and sense of achievement and support internal organi-zation.
5 Rhythmic: Brainstem-related rhythmic activities (including walking, running, rocking, dancing, drumming, singing, breathwork) prepare the brain for relational activities.
6 Respectful: Interventions must be respectful of the child, their family and their culture.

Keeping in mind the care needs of the typically developing child will provide clues to the needs of the child or adult who is struggling with a specific poorly developed brain region. Reflecting on the usual needs of a child who is organizing that brain region will assist the therapist to tailor their interventions to the appropriate developmental stage. It then becomes necessary to find a way to offer these interventions sequentially and in an age-appropriate way, so that they are acceptable, respectful and pleasurable for the client. Ongoing attention is paid to monitoring and co-regulating arousal state, so that the relationship is actively maintained during the activity.

For example, a client who is struggling with core state regulation and sensory integration, typically achieved in the first 2 years, will share some of the usual needs of an infant, who would typically benefit from:

- a calm, attentive, attuned adult providing assistance in learning to self-soothe and regulate behaviour;
- consistent, predictable physiological attention;
- routine;
- being held physically and emotionally;
- swaddling;
- slow, quiet, lilting speech and soothing sounds;
- rocking, gentle swinging, rhythmical movement;
- massage, patting;
- being soothed by experiences of being warm, safe, free from discomfort and satiated.

As the infant grows, new needs emerge, and they will typically enjoy (for example):

- being entertained by caregiver and responding to interactions by smiling, laughing, sharing attention, building anticipation;
- rhythmical, physical play with peaks of excitement (e.g. blowing raspberries, moving close and pulling back);
- playing peek-a-boo;
- playing with sound;
- playing with movement;
- exploration – first with eyes, then with hands, then with body;
- sensory and exploratory play.

It is possible to meet these needs even if they present in an adolescent or adult, but it is necessary to find ways to do this in an age-appropriate way, while remaining very alert to the optimal level of sensory arousal for the particular client. Early needs can be addressed by movement activities (ranging from physical play to Reiki), swinging in a hammock, safe massage (including hands, feet and head), gentle music, rhythmical drumming, bilateral stimulation, sensory play and Theraplay® activities. Age-appropriate musical, movement and dance interventions can be identified, for children, adolescents and adults, and will be explored in Chapters 5 and 6. Sensory and messy play and Theraplay activities (Munns, 2014), typically associated with infant and toddler play, are hugely important for those who have had difficult experiences in their early years. Chapter 7 explores ways to provide age-appropriate sensory-based interventions throughout the lifespan.

When choosing reparative experiences to address impairments in the limbic area and cortex (and to strengthen the vital neural network connecting these two regions), we consider the typical early childhood stages of development and experiences that usually assist the young child to achieve their developmental goals. In these years, children become more physically coordinated and skilled, make friends, learn to recognize and regulate their emotions, enhance both verbal and nonverbal communication, develop empathy and symbolic thinking, differentiate right from wrong and develop cognitive reasoning and problem-solving capacity. They benefit from social play and relationships; actively and experientially learning about their environment; play in its many forms (physical, exploratory, constructive, symbolic, sociodramatic, expressive, competitive etc.); developing coherent narratives and engaging with stories and performing arts; and formal education. Chapters 8–11 present a host of approaches, utilizing art, sand, storytelling, and dramatic and imaginative play, for use with clients throughout the lifetime to enhance limbic and cortical development and compensate for interruptions in their development and organization.

## Getting started

Even when working with clients whose development has not been seriously compromised, we are well advised (as indicated earlier with regard to the EPR model and both the 3 Rs and the 6 Rs) to pay attention to establishing safety at the beginning of the work. Gil (2013) points out that, when children begin therapy, it is highly likely that anxiety about coming has ensured that their brainstem is the most activated brain region, and they are likely to be experiencing anxiety, elevated pulse rate and altered breathing. In this situation, their cortex is not 'online', and there is no point in trying to engage them cognitively; their primary need is to calm down their regulatory system, and this will happen best in the context of relationship. Gil talks about useful engagement activities that are suited to this early stage: playing music or introducing drumming, telling a story that incorporates guided imagery, breathing activities, blowing bubbles or blowing up balloons. This sequential approach to introducing brain-based activities is targeting the lower brain region first to establish regulation.

When targeting this region, whether for a few moments at the start of a session, for some time during the session if a fear-based response is triggered in the child, or for a more prolonged period if the client is persistently unable to achieve state regulation because of a grossly dysfunctional stress response and a baseline state of alarm/fear, another consideration is to determine whether the client is hypo-aroused or hyperaroused. Some clients will lean more towards one of these, whereas others may swing in a disorganized fashion between them. What works for one client will not necessarily work for another, as each will have their own sensory profile that will also impact on their needs. The aim is to assist the client to achieve a balanced level of arousal and regulation.

The client who is hyperaroused and oversensitive to stimuli will benefit from down-regulating activities that inhibit their physiological responses by their utilizing physical effort and expending energy. These include all activities that involve structure, effort and working against a resistant medium, especially when including slow, rhythmical movement and/or familiar, predictable touch. Calming activities include deep-pressure, full-body activities such as pushing, pulling, hanging and crawling, lifting and carrying weights, digging sand or mud, throwing (at or into a target) and hands and upper-body-only activities (stirring, pressing, kneading, squeezing or pinching, e.g. clay, fidgeting with a toy that offers resistance) and activities requiring concentration (walking on balance beam). Mild flavours and calming oral activities such as sucking or blowing can be favoured. Soft, gentle, rhythmical sounds and music are also useful.

The client who is hypoaroused and under-responsive will seek out stimulation including strong tastes (sour, citrus, spicy, bitter) and smells, rough textures, contrasting images, uneven beats, alerting oral activities (sucking/chewing ice, eating chewy/crunchy food, licking, chewing toys), high-energy dabbing, poking, playful touch and fast-paced, jarring movements. They have poor body and boundary awareness and will benefit from playing in materials that encase them

Table 2.2 A neurodevelopmental approach to case conceptualization and treatment planning

| Hypothetical case details | Presenting issues | Potential impact on brain development | Neurodevelopmentally appropriate intervention |
|---|---|---|---|
| While pregnant, Lauren was physically and emotionally assaulted by her partner Paul. The abuse continued through to the birth, although Lauren did not report it for several months, by which time her baby, David, was 4 months old | Lauren generally has a low mood and minimal energy. She finds looking after David tiring. David is fed on demand and is always bathed and in clean clothing (in fact Lauren changes him many times a day). He does not sleep well, however, and is lower than average weight. He is fed on demand, but his appetite seems low. He cries often and loudly, and Lauren verbalizes difficulty in holding him, given his anticipated fearful or angry cries whether he is being held or left to cry in his crib | Trauma here may have impacted on the development of David's brain through the pregnancy owing to the stress Lauren was under. In addition, at this early age, brainstem development and the development of the diencephalon may have been impacted, these areas being associated with sleep and appetite | Lauren is meeting David's basic needs, but both Lauren and David would benefit from engagement in Theraplay, which promotes touch and interaction – peek-a-boo, nursery rhymes or singing games can encourage this. David may also benefit from sensory stimulation and baby massage. In the absence of Theraplay, a parenting skills programme/psycho-education focusing on the importance of touch and attunement would be beneficial |
| Ben was taken into care when he was 3 years old because of his mothers' active alcoholism. She lost her partner, Ben's father, soon after Ben's first birthday and, although she had not drunk for 4 years, she relapsed within 2 months of the funeral. Ben needs were no | Ben has started nursery school, and the staff at the children's centre have noticed that he spends much of his time observing what is going on rather than taking part in activities. He appears 'clumsy', his solitary play is exploratory – picking up toys, putting them into | Trauma here may have impacted on the development of Ben's brain at a number of levels, particularly the midbrain and delaying development of the limbic area. He appears to be presenting with difficulties associated with the limbic area, demonstrating issues with social | It might be useful for staff at the children's centre to be briefed about potential explanations for Ben's difficulties. In particular, discussion might focus on how trauma and the development of play are closely related, and that mastering early forms of play is needed before more complex play |

longer consistently met when his mum started drinking. For example, he was once left alone for 16 hours until neighbours were alerted by his crying and secured entry to care for him. At this point, the authorities became involved

his mouth, shaking and banging them and looking closely at them. He is easily distressed, rarely speaks to the staff or other children and avoids eye contact. Although his mum says he was a good sleeper as an infant, this is no longer true. He often rocks in his crib to self-soothe. During meal times, he will eat until he is sick, so caregivers need to ensure that he is provided with appropriate portions. He eats quickly and is always looking around to compare what he has with the meals of other children. He will refuse help from staff or his foster parents. He will run out of the centre if upset, but does not run to anywhere in particular. Music can be effective in soothing him

interaction and attachment. His under-developed play skills may be indicative of trauma associated with the midbrain

can evolve. Routine and the repetition of activities will facilitate a sense of trust and predictability. Within the centre, the sensory play that Ben frequently engages in can be expanded (playing with both dry and wet substances and a variety of textures) and encouraged, with opportunities added for social interaction within this play. Adults can bring an air of playfulness to shared activities. Gross motor play should also be facilitated. Development of the midbrain might be encouraged through music and movement, with a particular emphasis on rhythm and repetitive movements such as drumming or dance activities. Restricting the number of staff that he is negotiating and navigating relationships with will help him to begin to feel safe

*continued ...*

Table 2.2 Continued

| Hypothetical case details | Presenting issues | Potential impact on brain development | Neurodevelopmentally appropriate intervention |
|---|---|---|---|
| Antonia is an 11-year-old girl who is the second of four siblings. Though Antonia has lived in a loving adoptive home for 4 years, she previously lived in two other foster homes after being taken into care at the age of 5. Antonia's biological parents argued all the time. Mother had a substance abuse problem and moved to another part of the country, away from her husband but with her four children, to begin a new life. Antonia was often required to diaper and care for her younger twin siblings. Her older brother often watched pornographic television, and all the children observed their mother having relations with various men | Antonia's presenting problems appear to be a direct result of her early exposure to multiple complex trauma events, as well as lack of exposure to age-appropriate activities. Antonia's adoptive parents sought therapeutic intervention because Antonia appeared very disorganized, left messes everywhere, avoided family mealtimes, would not accept help from her parents and was very impulsive and easily angered. She wouldn't sleep in her own bed and was often observed to be self-harming after achieving low marks at school or being corrected at home. She had limited peer social skills and would isolate herself for long periods of time. Antonia has not developed a connection with her adoptive parents as yet, although she has been placed with them | Given that Antonia's play skills and emotional functioning do not match with her chronological age, and that her complex history is likely to have led to impairment in all areas of brain development, a comprehensive treatment plan is needed. This will include regular home-based interventions, plus therapist-directed and -facilitated play sessions, including self-directed play. Parental and therapist warmth and attunement to Antonia's emotional states will be important, as will simple tracking and reflective commentary. Interventions are intended to initially address the brainstem and midbrain area by focusing first on establishing state regulation through positive touch and repetitive sensory input. Music-, rhythm- and movement-based activities will increase somatosensory integration. | Antonia often functions emotionally at a level below that expected of an 11-year-old. Ascertaining and responding in a stage- (rather than age-) appropriate manner to her developmental functioning moment to moment will be important. Antonia needs assistance to get in touch with bodily sensations. A stethoscope will be shared with the family, with a plan for Antonia to first chart her resting heartbeat and then later her heartbeat when she is becoming agitated, so as to help her recognize when she needs parental assistance and calming activities. Hand or foot massages with baby lotion will help Antonia experience safe, nurturing touch. Routines and repetition of activities in her school and home-life spaces will provide consistency and predictability for Antonia. Relaxation exercises and playing |

for 4 years. They report that she often attempts to play them off against each other in order to be the person in the house who is in control. She approaches the parent who took parenting leave more readily. Antonia has broken many items around the home in anger, including items that are special to her. Antonia has difficulty maintaining focus and attention. Projects and assignments are often unfinished or not handed in to her teacher when they are complete. Her teacher describes her as being hyperactive and hypervigilant. She has been reported to struggle with transitions both at school and home. She becomes aggressive when she has to wait to get attention or to have a need met

Antonia's needs in these areas are indicated by her lack of regulation, hypervigilance and persistent anxiety. Later interventions will address limbic system deficiencies to improve emotional regulation and tolerance through art, play and social activities. Finally, story-based and dramatic activities will support cortical development and improve and increase Antonia's capacity for abstract thinking and insight (Perry, 2006)

relaxing music may help Antonia to self-soothe at bedtime. Antonia will benefit from a combination of Theraplay and non-directive play therapy sessions. Her adoptive parents can be part of these sessions at key times. When the interventions at home and school and in play therapy sessions show evidence of assisting brainstem and midbrain functioning, Antonia may be ready for limbic- and cortical-oriented approaches that include art-based, drama-based and narrative work, as well as bibliotherapy. This will include activities that focus on turn-taking and sharing. Expressive and creative materials such as art supplies, dressing-up clothes, puppets and sandtray will be provided, as will games with rules. The therapist could present a trauma training workshop so that school staff can understand that Antonia's behaviour is often a coping style based on trauma history

Howard et al., 2014. Reproduced with permission from Routledge (e.g. hammocks, tunnels, lycra suits). Up-regulating activities to encourage exploration and ignite curiosity and playfulness include large, free movements, unstructured dance, spinning, swinging, running, bouncing and working against gravity (including hanging upside down).

Table 2.2 presents three short hypothetical cases with details of life events, and associated timing, that compromised the child's development, potential impact on brain development, presenting issues and suggested neurodevelopmentally appropriate interventions.

## The other 23 hours

Therapy sessions are only one element in responding to the therapeutic and developmental needs of clients with complex needs. Sessions are traditionally scheduled for one hour per week, and a resourcing stage will be our priority in the early stages of intervention. This is an important component in a client's healing and in supporting them to develop strategies to self-regulate. However, we also need to pay close attention to finding ways to support healing and a capacity to remain grounded in all situations, not just the therapy room. When we are working with vulnerable clients, this includes a number of components to build the client's own resources and, particularly with young clients, working with family members and other supportive allies who can assist them in maintaining regulation or regaining a state of calmness when stressed or inappropriately triggered (Fraser, 2014). As described above, clients can learn a number of strategies to assist them in self-regulating and inhibiting inappropriate arousal states in nurturing and fun ways. A psycho-educational component is useful to enable all involved to understand the relevant physiology and interpersonal neurobiological context.

When the client is dependent on others because of their age and/or developmental status, it is beneficial to explore options of working with others within their homes and perhaps other significant environments (e.g. school) to develop a supportive, attuned, enriching and developmentally responsive system. In essence, parents/ carers and other adults in the child's world can become part of the child's resources, to enhance healthy coping and facilitate them in up-regulating or down-regulating as necessary. Many adult clients will also welcome some joint sessions with important people in their lives so that they can strengthen their supportive network. The provision of support to caregivers and partners can ensure that they feel held, confident and capable, and are empowered by the role ascribed to them. Working in partnership is of critical importance in providing for safety, consistency and repetitive positive experiences.

Psycho-educational inputs will include a focus on developing an understanding of trauma and recovery. Appropriate family members will benefit from learning to attune to the client's level of arousal and sense of safety, so that they can be of assistance in co-regulation or in helping them to use self-regulation strategies. An inability to engage playfully or seek appropriate care and comfort indicates that the client's brain may be in a state of fear-related activation, and they may need help to connect with a trusted person and thereby reduce their impulsivity and regain self-control. This will include a heightened awareness of the client's hypervigilance and preoccupation with nonverbal cues that will remind the support person to move slowly when the client's fear system is activated. Some useful strategies include dropping to the child's level, smiling, giving eye contact, touching gently and modelling slow, deep breathing with a focus on the out breath. If words are necessary, speak quietly and slowly. Murmuring and motherese may be more appropriate than words. Having other strategies to hand – for example, blowing bubbles, safe-place visualization, sensory play materials, soft music, rhythmic movement, physical relaxation activity, progressive muscle relaxation, a self-talk line or any activity that will assist the client to make a deeper connection with the here and now – will be useful. A good match between the client's interest and tolerance and the intervention is important!

Carers will also be invested in trying to prevent the child getting triggered into alarm states as much as possible. This will involve them in providing routines, being predictable, being nurturing and comforting, reading the child's nonverbal cues and assisting them to learn language to express their needs, offering an appropriate number and type of choice. Providing appropriate boundaries will support the child in learning to inhibit impulses. Learning to intervene to distract or to terminate activities that are triggering the child is an important skill. Providing training in non-directive, reflective language is particularly useful, so that the adult is equipped to provide supportive language responses to whatever is immediately engaging the child. Giving language to immediate experiences enhances the child's emotional vocabulary, supports the development of neural pathways between lower and higher brain regions and connects the right and left hemispheres in ways that enhance processing of previously unresolved material.

Our aim as therapists and the hopes of our young clients and their caregivers are likely to be the same: to reach a stage where behaviour is adaptive to the current environment and the social engagement system is functioning fully. Porges tells us that, 'once we can easily engage the social engagement system, we are free to mobilize without being in fight or flight. Rather than fight or flight, we can move and play' (2011: 14). Not only that: we can live more fully, experience more positive emotions and engage in more satisfying, spontaneous relationships.

## Key points

- Neurobiological evidence supports the integration of play and creative arts approaches into a neurosequential approach to psychotherapy with clients throughout the lifespan.
- The starting point for therapy is to modulate the primary regulatory networks; later interventions will sequentially address the disorganized brain regions of the specific client.

- Determining if the client is hypoaroused or hyperaroused will assist the therapist in choosing appropriate up-regulating or down-regulating interventions.
- Effective therapy work with child clients generally requires the active involvement of their carers.

## References

Badenoch, B., and Kestly, T. (2015). Exploring the neuroscience of healing play at every age. In A.L. Stewart and D.A. Crenshaw (eds) *Play Therapy: A comprehensive guide to theory and practice* (pp. 524–38). New York: Guilford Press.

Bratton, S., Ray, D., Rhide, T., and Jones, L. (2005). The efficacy of play therapy with children: A meta-analytic review of treatment outcomes. *Professional Psychology: Research & Practice, 36*, 378–90.

Brown, S., and Vaughan, C. (2009). *Play: How it shapes the brain, opens the imagination, and invigorates the soul.* New York: Avery.

Carey, L. (2006). *Expressive and Creative Arts Methods for Trauma Survivors.* London: Jessica Kingsley.

Fraser, T. (2014). How neuroscience can inform play therapy practice with parents and children. In E. Prendiville and J. Howard (eds) *Play Therapy Today: Contemporary practice for individuals, groups, and parents* (pp. 179–98). London: Routledge.

Gaskill, R., and Perry, B.D. (2014). The neurobiological power of play: Using the neurosequential model of therapeutics to guide play in the healing process. In C. Malchiodi and D.A. Crenshaw (eds) *Play and Creative Arts Therapy for Attachment Trauma* (pp. 178–94). New York: Guilford Press.

Gil, E. (2006). *Helping Abused and Traumatized Children: Integrating directive and nondirective approaches.* New York: Guilford Press.

Gil, E. (2010). *Working with Children to Heal Interpersonal Trauma.* New York: Guilford Press.

Gil, E. (2013). Integrating a neurosequential approach in the treatment of traumatized children. Interview with C.F. Sori and S. Schnur. *The Family Journal: Counseling & Therapy for Couples & Families.* DOI: 10.1177/1066480713514945.

Green, E., and Drewes, A. (2014). *Integrating Expressive Arts and Play Therapy with Children and Adolescents: A guidebook for mental health practitioners and educators.* Hoboken, NJ: Wiley.

Howard, J., Prendiville, E., and Fraser, T. (2014). A neurodevelopmental approach to case conceptualization and treatment planning. In E. Prendiville and J. Howard (eds) *Play Therapy Today: Contemporary practice for individuals, groups, and parents* (pp. 191–5). London: Routledge.

Jennings, S. (1999). *An Introduction to Developmental Playtherapy.* London: Jessica Kingsley.

Jennings, S. (2011). *Healthy Attachments and Neuro-Dramatic-Play.* London: Jessica Kingsley.

Jennings, S. (2014). Applying an Embodiment–Projection–Role framework in groupwork with children. In E. Prendiville and J. Howard (eds) *Play Therapy Today: Contemporary practice for individuals, groups, and parents* (pp. 81–96). London: Routledge.

MacKinnon, L. (2012). The neurosequential model of therapeutics: An interview with Bruce Perry. *Australian & New Zealand Journal of Family Therapy*, *33*(3), 210–18.

Malchiodi, C.A. (2014). Neurobiology, creative interventions and childhood trauma. In C. Malchiodi (ed) *Creative Interventions with Traumatized Children* (2nd edn, pp. 3–23). New York: Guilford Press.

Malchiodi, C.A., and Crenshaw, D.A. (eds) (2014). *Creative Arts and Play Therapy for Attachment Problems*. New York: Guilford Press.

Munns, E. (2014). Group Theraplay. In E. Prendiville and J. Howard (eds) *Play Therapy Today: Contemporary practice for individuals, groups, and parents* (pp. 163–78). London: Routledge.

Perry, B.D. (2006). The neurosequential model of therapeutics: Applying principles of neuroscience to clinical work with traumatized and maltreated children. In N.B. Webb (ed.) *Working with Traumatized Youth in Child Welfare* (pp. 27–52). New York: Guilford Press.

Perry, B.D., and Hambrick, E.P. (2008). The neurosequential model of therapeutics. *Reclaiming Children & Youth*, *17*(3): 38–43.

Porges, S.W. (2011). *The Polyvagal Theory: Neurophysiological foundations of emotions, attachment, communication, self regulation*. New York: Norton.

Schaefer, C.E., and Drewes, A. (2014). *The Therapeutic Powers of Play: 20 core agents of change* (2nd edn). Hoboken, NJ: Wiley.

van der Kolk, B.A. (2003). The neurobiology of childhood trauma and abuse. *Child & Adolescent Psychiatric Clinics*, *12*, 293–317.

Chapter 3

# The role of non-directive and directive/focused approaches to play and expressive arts therapy for children, adolescents, and adults

Terry Kottman, Rebecca Dickinson
and Kristin Meany-Walen

There are many approaches to play therapy and expressive arts that can be used in the therapeutic treatment of children, adolescents, and adults (Nash and Schaefer, 2011; Drewes and Bratton, 2014; Graves-Alcorn and Green, 2014; Frey, 2015; Gardner, 2015). These approaches range along a continuum from non-directive to focused/directive (Yasenik and Gardner, 2012). This chapter is designed to introduce play therapy and expressive arts therapies to professionals new to the field and to provide clarity about the various approaches to play therapy and expressive arts therapies for more experienced practitioners.

Play therapy is "the systematic use of a theoretical model to establish an interpersonal process wherein trained play therapists use the therapeutic powers of play to help clients prevent or resolve psychosocial difficulties and achieve optimal growth and development" (Association for Play Therapy, 2014, para 6). According to Schaefer and Drewes (2014), the therapeutic powers of play include facilitating communication (self-expression, access to the unconscious, direct teaching, and indirect teaching); fostering emotional wellness (catharsis, abreaction, positive emotions, counterconditioning fears, stress inoculation, and stress management); enhancing social relationships (therapeutic relationship, attachment formation, social competence, and empathy); and increasing personal strengths (creative problem solving, resiliency, moral development, accelerated psychological development, self-regulation and self-esteem). According to the British Association for Play Therapy (2014), play therapy is used with children, adolescents, adults, and families to relieve intra- and interpersonal difficulties through the use of creative modalities. Play therapy is used in a variety of settings that might include schools, private practices, community agencies, residential settings, and hospitals. Creative arts therapies consist of the intentional use of visual arts, dance/movement, music, and dramatic enactment, "within a psychotherapeutic framework. Like play therapy, they are experiential, active approaches that capitalize on engaging individuals of all ages in multisensory experiences for self-exploration, personal communication, developmental objectives, socialization, and emotional reparation" (Malchiodi, 2014: 3).

This chapter provides readers with a basic description of selected theoretical approaches to play therapy and selected forms of expressive arts therapy. The theoretical approaches to play therapy range from approaches that are consistently non-directive (child-centred, filial therapy, and Jungian), through approaches that are sometimes focused/directive and sometimes non-directive (Adlerian, cognitive behavioral, Gestalt, narrative, and psychodynamic), to the most focused/directive (Theraplay). Readers will find descriptions of the basic tenets, goals of therapy, intervention techniques and research for each of these approaches to play therapy. Information regarding the rationale for using expressive arts in therapy and descriptions of specific expressive arts approaches, including art therapy, music therapy, dance and movement therapy, and drama therapy, will also be provided. Readers are encouraged to seek out information from primary authors, provided in each description of a particular approach, for a more thorough analysis of individual approaches.

## Non-directive approaches to play therapy

### Child-centred play therapy

Virginia Axline (1947, 1964, 1969) was the first to write about child-centred play therapy (CCPT). This approach is based on Roger's person-centred theory, which views people as rational, positive, and with an innate tendency to heal, grow, mature, and self-actualize (Wilson and Ryan, 2005; Ray, 2011; Landreth, 2012). As the name implies, CCPT is usually conducted with children, but can be appropriate for adolescents as well. Ryan and Wilson (2005) suggested this approach can help adolescents "integrate into their developing sense of unique personal identity their earlier childhood experience, present concerns, and more adult concerns about the future" (p. 96).

According to CCPT, children are born with an organismic valuing system. Over time, children begin to internalize messages they receive from others and develop "conditions of worth," which are the qualities children believe they need to possess in order to receive love and feel valuable. The discrepancy between people's beliefs about their "real self" and their "ideal self" creates incongruence and, essentially, problems in the children's lives (VanFleet et al., 2010; Ray and Landreth, 2015).

Child-centred play therapists are non-directive and only engage in the child's play when they are invited to play by the child. They use play therapy skills of tracking, restating content, reflecting feeling, returning responsibility, setting limits, and using the whisper technique. In CCPT, the client moves through three stages (Sweeney and Landreth, 2009). During the first stage, the client is engaged in self-exploration. Here, clients examine where they are in their lives. Next, they begin to understand the relationship between where they are in life and where they would like to be in life. In the last phase, clients develop a plan for reducing the incongruence between their "real self" and their "ideal self." The child moves through these stages without direction from the counselor. CCPT counselors believe in the internal power of the child and the child's ability to lead the session in a meaningful and healing direction. The relationship, one of unconditional positive regard, empathy, and genuineness on the part of the counselor, is necessary and sufficient for positive client change. The core belief of CCPT in the importance of the relationship between the child and therapist is one of the foundational elements of the neurosequential model, in that it allows the child to engage in somatosensory activities without having to use language, which will set the stage for the facilitation of emotional regulation.

Numerous randomized control trials, single case research designs, and quasi-experimental studies have been conducted to support CCPT's efficacy with children who present with a range of concerns, such as academic problems (e.g. Blanco *et al.*, 2012), internalizing problems (e.g. Garza and Bratton, 2005), and externalizing/disruptive behaviors (e.g. Schottelkorb and Ray, 2009). Meta-analyses have also been conducted throughout the past few decades that strengthen the support for CCPT as an evidenced-based practice, demonstrating moderate-to-large effect sizes for internalizing behavior problems and externalizing behavior problems (e.g. Bratton *et al.*, 2005; Lin and Bratton, 2015).

## *Filial therapy*

Filial therapy (FT) operates as a psycho-educational model in which the therapist acts as an educator and coach in helping parents conduct non-directive play sessions with their own child. FT relies on the stages of non-directive play therapy in regards to the child's progression towards the therapeutic goals and follows Axline's principles of non-directive CCPT. FT was developed by Doctors Bernard and Louise Guerney (1987) in the 1950s and 1960s and has garnered strong research support as a play therapy intervention. It has been adapted into various other formats, including child–parent relationship therapy by Landreth and Bratton (2006).

Although there are direct goals in this therapeutic approach for both the child and parent/caregiver (VanFleet, 2003), the overarching goal is to strengthen familial relationships and, in turn, improve family functioning. Working with parents, filial therapists utilize a four-stage model after the initial assessment and observation of a play session between the child and parent. The first stage involves the therapist conducting a play session demonstration with the child, in which the parent observes the therapist utilizing the skills they will be learning. The second stage involves parent training of four essential skills: structuring, empathic listening, child-centred imaginary play, and limit-setting. The parent practices these skills through mock play sessions in which the therapist acts as the child and provides opportunities for the parent to try out these skills. There is a focus on encouraging and reinforcing the parent's progression in developing his or her skills, as well as recognizing and validating the parent's concerns about the process. When the parent has made progress in implementing the skills in mock sessions, the family moves on to the third stage, in which the therapist observes the parent engaging in non-directive play sessions with the child. After each play session, the parent and therapist engage in processing the play session, both from the parent's perspective and the therapist's. During these feedback sessions, the therapist begins teaching a new skill of interpreting the child's play themes, with the focus of helping the parent recognize alternative interpretations, rather than trying to determine definitive explanations. After multiple play sessions observed by the therapist, the family moves to conducting play sessions at home, with regular meetings between parent and therapist to process the play sessions. During this stage, the therapist begins helping the parent generalize the skills learned to situations outside the non-directive play sessions.

FT has a substantial amount of empirical support spanning 50 years and, as documented by VanFleet (2014), is one of the most researched forms of play therapy. A meta-analysis by Bratton *et al.* (2005) provided support that the effectiveness of play therapy is enhanced by involvement of parents, particularly through FT. In repeated studies, FT has been shown to improve child behaviors and presenting problems, parent empathy and acceptance, parent skill levels, parent stress, and satisfaction with family life (VanFleet *et al.*, 2005). Research has supported its use with a myriad of child and family issues across settings and cultures. FT has been used successfully with children who have trauma- or attachment-related issues, including with foster and adoptive families (VanFleet, 2014). With recognition of the effects of trauma on development, FT can be tailored for use with clients whose chronological age is much older than that for which the original model was designed, essentially meeting clients at the level they are at in order to improve functioning in familial relationships.

FT was used as the therapy model in two small studies by Barfield *et al.* (2012) on the neurosequential model with preschoolers. FT was specifically used to help the preschool staff develop an empathic environment in which the children felt understood and accepted. This empathic environment was used as the backdrop for the structured somatosensory activities from the neurosequential model. Although small samples were used, the two small studies supported the combined use of FT with the neurosequential model (Barfield *et al.*, 2012).

### *Jungian play therapy*

Jungian play therapy, popularized by J.P. Lilly, J. Allan, and E. Green, is grounded in Carl Jung's theoretical constructs. Jungian play therapy holds that, as children develop, the Self separates from the ego, creating individuation and uniqueness. Reintegration of the Self and the ego is a lifelong process and one that includes the integration of a person's psychic bipolarities. Jungians describe people creating archetypes, unconscious symbols that hold spiritual energy and feelings associated with their unique cultures, from their own phenomenological perspective. The symbols might appear in dreams, fantasies, and creative play, such as a wise old owl or a steady horse (Green, 2009, 2011). A central component of Jungian play therapy is the *collective unconscious*, which is an archetype that transcends people across cultures and eras.

People encounter intrapersonal or interpersonal difficulties when their real or perceived needs are not met. With needs not met, people create strategies that keep themselves psychologically safe (Allan, 1997). This might include denial, repression, projection, introjection, over-inflation, or anxiety. To repair the potential nascent functioning, the Jungian play therapist is an observer–participant, using directive and non-directive techniques (Green, 2009, 2011; Lilly, 2015). He or she creates an emotionally safe environment in which the counselor honors the images chosen by clients.

The Jungian play therapy process follows multiple stages and is customized for individual clients. First, the play therapist builds a nurturing and safe environment where the client can feel good enough. Next, the client freely expresses difficult emotions through play or other creative strategies. The third step allows the client to give attention to his or her rage, so that it can be processed and changed. The play therapist might also work with parents, teachers, family members, or communities to help the client thought the healing process. The ultimate goal is for clients to identify and activate their self-healing archetypes (Green, 2009, 2011; Lilly, 2015). When this happens, the client can begin to integrate the different parts of his or her personality, creating a more unified personality.

Similar to the other non-directive approaches to play therapy, the relationship with the child can create a situation in which the child can use somatosensory activities in the process of developing a sense of self-regulation. Many Jungian play therapists encourage regressive, foundational play that is an important component of the neurosequential model (Gaskill and Perry, 2014).

## Focused/directive approaches to play therapy

### Theraplay

Theraplay was developed by Ann Jernberg in the 1960s. Jernberg (1979) was heavily influenced by Bowlby's attachment theory, as well as interpersonal theories, including Kohut's self psychology theory and Winnicott's object relations theory (Booth and Jernberg, 2010; Booth and Winstead, 2015). The emphasis in these theories is on the importance of the parent–infant relationship, which forms a template for later relationships and interactional styles. "Theraplay advocates going back to that first relationship to make it a healthier one, through replicating what normal parents do with a young child" (Munns, 2011: 276). Theraplay matches well with neurosequential research and theory in the understanding the effect of stress and trauma on brain development in early childhood (Munns, 2011). Theraplay therapists strive to meet the client's developmental stage, which can be significantly younger than his or her chronological age. Attachment theory research also provides support to Theraplay in regards to how attachment patterns develop and persist through life. The soothing and nurturing that a client receives in a Theraplay session seeks to enhance the development of the right hemisphere of the brain to promote emotional regulation (Booth and Jernberg, 2010; Munns, 2011).

Theraplay is a focused/directive and structured form of play therapy where the aim is to heal attachment issues rooted in early childhood and to strengthen relationships (Booth and Jernberg, 2010; Munns, 2011). The basic principles of Theraplay hold that the therapy process should be (a) interactive and relationship-based; (b) direct and here-and-now focused; (c) guided by the adult (first the therapist and later the parent); (d) filled with attunement, empathy, responsiveness, and reflection; (e) focused on preverbal, social and right-brain activities; (f) multi-sensory, with an emphasis on touching; and (g) playful (Booth and Winstead, 2015). Although most of the literature features work with children and adolescents, Theraplay always includes parents or caretakers as co-therapists, which effectively includes adults as clients in the Theraplay process, and it can also be used with family groups and groups of adults (Munns, 2014).

The therapist provides directed interventions, based on the client's needs, as a vehicle for promoting attachment, trust, engagement with others, and self-esteem. Attention is also given to promoting self-regulation of emotions by structuring activities to avoid over-stimulation. The therapist plays the lead role in all sessions. Parents are often included in later sessions and are encouraged to take more of an active role as therapy progresses, and the therapist guides the parents in attuning to their child.

Assessment includes an intake interview with parents and the Marschak Interaction Method (Munns, 2011; Booth and Winstead, 2015). Interventions are designed based on the individual needs of clients, parents, and family members. Theraplay activities are categorized into four dimensions: structure (creating a sense of security and safety), engagement (creating connection between adult and child), nurture (creating feelings of calmness and being cared for), and challenge (creating age-appropriate risks where the child can be successful). Theraplay is typically a short-term intervention model lasting about eighteen sessions, but longer durations in treatment can be utilized for more severe attachment issues. Once underlying attachment issues are addressed in Theraplay, it is often possible to address other behavioral and emotional issues through a referral to other play therapy services.

Research on Theraplay is growing, with research increasingly including pre- and post comparisons between control and treatment groups (Munns, 2011; Booth and Jernberg, 2015). Research thus far supports Theraplay's therapeutic benefits in three areas: improved self-esteem, improved attachment, and lower aggression levels. Research that has included control groups has demonstrated improvements in self-esteem (Siu, 2009) and social skills (Siu, 2014), reduction in oppositional behavior (Wettig et al., 2006), increased empathy in teenage mothers (Ammen, 2000), and improvements in assertiveness, self-confidence, and trust (Wettig et al., 2011). Research on Theraplay has been conducted around the world in a variety of cultural contexts and has supported the application of Theraplay across cultures.

## Approaches to play therapy that are sometimes focused/directive and sometimes non-directive

### Adlerian play therapy

Adlerian play therapy was developed by Terry Kottman in the late 1980s and aligns with the teachings of Adler's individual psychology. Currently, it is one of the most commonly used approaches to play therapy in the United States (Lambert *et al.*, 2007). In Adlerian play therapy, therapists often work with children, adolescents, adults, and families. When working with children and adolescents, parent (and teacher, when appropriate) consultation is an integral part of the process of play therapy.

Adlerian play therapy is based on the assumptions that people are socially embedded and strive to find significance and belonging in the social world, are self-determined and creative, and perceive reality subjectively (Kottman and Ashby, 2015; Kottman and Meany-Walen, in press). People usually develop their lifestyles—the general orientation toward life and relationships—before the age of 6–8. Because youngsters are often egocentric, they may believe that things that occur in their lives are somehow about or because of them. This tendency can lead to misperceptions children incorporate into their lifestyles in the form of basic convictions about self, others, and the world (Griffith and Powers, 2007). These misperceptions and misinterpretations evolve into a system of "mistaken" beliefs—self-defeating and discouraged ideas about self, others, and the world. Regardless of the accuracy of these beliefs, people act as if they are true; their conscious and unconscious behaviors stem from those beliefs and are designed to help them gain significance and belonging.

In conceptualizing clients, Adlerian play therapists consider their assets; family constellation/birth order; family atmosphere; crucial Cs (courage, connect, capable, count; Lew and Bettner, 2000); personality priorities (pleasing, comfort, control, and superiority); goals of misbehaviors (attention, power, revenge, and proving inadequacy); life tasks (work/school, friends, family/intimacy, self, spirituality); and beliefs about self, others, and the world (Kottman, 2009; Kottman and Ashby, 2015; Kottman and Meany-Walen, in press). Adlerian play therapists work to help clients readjust their thinking, feeling, and behaving. Therapeutic goals include promoting social interest, decreasing feelings of inferiority and learning healthier ways of dealing with them, overcoming discouragement, recognizing assets and resources, changing mistaken beliefs, moving toward positive manifestations of personality priorities, mastering the crucial Cs, and mastering life tasks.

Adlerian play therapists employ focused/directive and non-directive strategies throughout the play therapy process (Kottman and Meany-Walen, in press). Play therapy skills used in Adlerian play therapy include generic skills used in many approaches to play therapy (e.g. tracking, restating content, reflecting feelings, returning responsibility, limit-setting) and skills that are specific to Adlerian play therapy (e.g. metacommunicating, encouraging, spitting in the client's soup—

which is simply pointing out when the client is doing something self-defeating). Adlerian play therapists also use strategies that might include sandtray, art techniques, role-plays, bibliotherapy, movement and dance, and creation of therapeutic metaphors. Interventions are custom-designed, with the aim of helping clients to gain insight and/or practice new, more socially useful ways of feeling, thinking, and/or behaving.

Adlerian play therapy is comprised of four phases of therapy: building an egalitarian relationship between the therapist and the client, exploring the client's lifestyle, helping the client gain insight, and reorienting/re-educating the client (Kottman and Meany-Walen, in press). In the first phase, the play therapist and client work to build a therapeutic relationship in which there is shared power and trust. During the next phase, the play therapist allows for free play and creates games or interventions to gather information about the client and the client's lifestyle. In the third phase, the play therapist designs interventions to help the client understand how his or her thinking, feeling, and/or behaving might be getting in the way of healthy functioning. Last, the client and play therapist rehearse and evaluate new, more effective ways of finding significance and belonging in the world.

Throughout the process of Adlerian play therapy, the child is often encouraged to engage in play such as dance, music-making, movement, and art, which, according to the neurosequential model, can encourage somatosensory integration and facilitate emotional regulation. In the later phases of the process, the therapist helps foster abstract thinking by engaging the child in storytelling, drama, and art activities.

Empirical research supporting the efficacy of Adlerian play therapy has recently gained momentum. A growing body of research has been published that supports the effectiveness of Adlerian play therapy, particularly with children who have externalizing, problematic behaviors (e.g. Akay, 2013; Meany-Walen *et al.*, 2014, 2015, in press; Dillman Taylor and Meany-Walen, 2015).

## *Cognitive behavioral play therapy*

Cognitive behavioral therapy (CBT), developed by Aaron Beck, was adapted by Susan Knell (1993) into cognitive behavioral play therapy (CBPT) in the 1990s. CBPT is a psycho-educational model that provides developmentally appropriate therapy interventions to children based on the original concepts of CBT (Knell and Dasari, 2009; Knell, 2011; Cavett, 2015). It is a focused approach to play therapy in which the therapist utilizes intentional interventions aimed at reaching therapeutic goals, often employing modelling and role-playing through playful interactions. The process is directive, structured, and goal-directed. Although Knell designed CBPT for children, it easily could be applied to adolescents and adults, as the root interventions of CBT were initially developed for adults.

This approach to play therapy is based on the tenet that the way individuals structure and interpret experiences determines their emotions and behavior

(Knell, 1993, 2011). In other words, what one thinks determines how one feels and acts. A person's schemas (core beliefs and basic assumptions) have an important impact on how he or she operates cognitively. At times, a person's beliefs and assumptions can predispose him or her to psychological distress.

In CBPT, the focus for the therapeutic process is on changing the child's thoughts, feelings, beliefs, fantasies, and environment (Knell, 1993, 2011; Knell and Dasari, 2009; Cavett, 2015). The goal in therapy is to help the child develop more adaptive thoughts, beliefs, and behaviors. The process of CBPT has four stages: assessment, introduction/orientation, middle stage (focused on interventions), and preparation for termination. Parent consultation, in which the play therapist actually teaches parents cognitive and behavioral strategies for supporting the work done in play therapy sessions, is an essential element in CBPT.

Although the relationship between client and therapist is considered important, it is not considered to be the primary catalyst for change (Knell, 1993, 2011; Knell and Dasari, 2009). The most important intervention strategies in CBPT (done with art materials, puppets, and figures) are modeling, role-playing, semi-structured play (in which the therapist sets up scenarios for puppets or figures who need the client's help to "solve their problems"), cognitive restructuring, positive self-statements, bibliotherapy, problem-solving skills, relaxation training, systematic desensitization, contingency management, stimulus fading, and extinction (Knell and Dasari, 2009).

CBT has a long history of empirical support regarding its effectiveness with adults in treating depression, anxiety, and phobias, and there are studies designed to demonstrate the efficacy of trauma-focused CBT with children (Hoch, 2009) and game-based CBT (Springer and Misurell, 2012). These are not specifically CBPT, and so more research is needed to demonstrate the efficacy of these interventions as part of CBPT (Knell, 2011). One study specifically designed to research the efficacy of CBPT was a study involving Iranian preschool children, in which researchers using CBPT found a significant reduction in emotional and behavioral symptoms (Jafari *et al.*, 2011).

## *Gestalt play therapy*

Gestalt play therapy has been a respected approach to play therapy for several decades. Violet Oaklander (1978/1992) developed Gestalt play therapy, which has its roots in Perls' Gestalt psychology. Wellness and mental health are deemed a product of a person's ability to act and react as a total organism and to self-regulate within his or her environment. Ideally, a person integrates all aspects of his or her being, which includes senses, physical body, emotions, and cognitions, and moves through life with intention and awareness and is free to continue to develop and change throughout life (Carroll, 2009; Oaklander, 2011). Problems occur when a person creates fragments or compartments of his or her being, or when he or she distributes concentration and attention among several areas simultaneously. He or she may not grasp the influence he or she has on the environment and the influence the environment has on him- or herself. The person becomes stagnant or stuck in particular patterns of relating to the environment. This process is usually created with the intention of survival and maintaining optional functioning and is typically out of the person's awareness (Carroll, 2009; Oaklander, 2011). A primary goal of Gestalt play therapy is for the client to work through and integrate the unfinished business that creates feelings of *stuckness* in the person's life. Gestalt play therapy is usually used with children, but can be appropriate for adolescents and adults as well.

The Gestalt play therapist can be either non-directive or directive, depending on the child, the stage of therapy, the presenting problem(s), and the material the child brings to a particular session (Carroll, 2009; Oaklander, 2011). The therapist provides nurture and support that allow the client to engage in the counseling process and become more fully aware and accepting of him- or herself as a unique, whole, and creative being. Gestalt play therapists will conduct "experiments" with clients with the goal of increasing clients' total organismic awareness. The experiment is an opportunity in the therapy session for the client to try something with the goal of simply seeing what happens. Other play therapy skills include reflecting feelings, using art techniques, role-playing, reading books or watching movies, moving and movement activities, and using projective techniques and interpretations (Carroll, 2009; Oaklander, 1978/1992, 2006).

Following the initial building of the relationship, Gestalt play therapy treatment stages are individualized to the client and the client's needs (Carroll, 2009). The play therapist works with the client and the client's social support system to develop an understanding of the client's functioning and areas that might be causing distress to the client. The counselor respects that the client's history and the restoration of his or her organismic self-regulation will unfold in a time and manner necessary for the client (Oaklander, 2006). This process cannot be hurried or slowed. Termination occurs as the client and the client's social supports (if applicable) indicate better functioning in the client's different environments (Carroll, 2009).

Gestalt play therapy could be used in conjunction with the neurosequential model, using the client–therapist relationship as the foundation for the work and building directive and/or experimental activities into sessions to encourage somatosensory integration through movement and music-making and dance, play and art to facilitate emotional regulation. In later sessions, the Gestalt play therapist would use storytelling, drama activities, and art techniques to help foster the client's abstract thinking processes. Gestalt fits well with the neurosequential model in its individualized approach to each client's needs.

### *Narrative play therapy*

There are several different approaches to narrative play therapy (Cattanach, 2008; Mills, 2015). Ann Cattanach (2006, 2008) adapted one form of narrative play therapy from Michael White's narrative therapy model, which involves the therapist asking the client questions as a means of developing vivid descriptions of life experiences. Joyce Mills (2015) developed a different approach to narrative play therapy, called StoryPlay, based on the work of Milton Erickson, in which the therapist uses both the client's symptoms and the client's story to "evoke behavioral and emotional transformational change" (Mills, 2015: 171).

In both approaches to narrative play therapy, sometimes the therapist follows the client's lead, and other times the therapist leads the client. The narrative play therapist allows the client to direct many of their interactions, but, in Cattanach's version, the therapist utilizes a curious and genuine approach in questioning the client to help the client develop his or her narrative and explore alternative endings (Cattanach, 2006). The therapist also has the role of recording the narratives as they emerge. In both versions, the client is free to create a narrative through a variety of options, including using toys, props, and sensory materials. The therapist and client co-construct the narrative through the therapeutic activities, dialogue, and relationship (Cattanach, 2008; Mills and Crowley, 2014). The therapist also provides stories for the client that are relevant to the client's narrative themes, including culturally based as well as published stories and legends. The goal in both versions of narrative play therapy is to help the client develop a new, more adaptive life story. In both versions, the client can be a child, an adolescent or an adult.

The neurosequential model of brain development supports the therapeutic relationship used in narrative play therapy to help the child progress to higher levels of reasoning, as well as supporting the value of play to helping the client develop a greater sense of self-awareness and well-being (Taylor de Faoite, 2011).

## *Psychodynamic play therapy*

Psychodynamic play therapy is the oldest approach to play therapy. Early practitioners of psychoanalytic/psychodynamic play therapy included Hug-Hellmuth (1921), who was the first author to write about using play in therapy with children, Anna Freud (1946), who used play as a tool for building relationships with children in therapy, and Klein (1932), who considered child's play to be the equivalent of the verbal expression that takes place in adult psychotherapy. Historically, most psychodynamic play therapists have worked with children (Lee, 2009; Levy, 2011; Mordock, 2015).

In psychodynamic play therapy, the focus is on identifying and resolving unconscious conflicts that are driving psychological symptoms. The psychodynamic play therapist explores clients' feelings and how they lead them to exhibit problematic behaviors, which are thought to be indicative of deeper, underlying struggles (Crenshaw, 2008; Mordock, 2015). Through the psychodynamic lens, the maladaptive behaviors are defense mechanisms designed to protect the psyche from unpleasant consequences of these conflicts. Through play, the clients work through the unconscious material and resolve the intra-psychic conflicts that interfere with their development (Lee, 2009; Levy, 2011). Clients unconsciously project life experiences and relationships on to the play materials. This process facilitates change through catharsis and labelling feelings, having corrective emotional experiences, working through conflict, learning coping techniques, cultivating insight, and developing internal structure (Crenshaw, 2008; Kottman, 2011; Mordock, 2015).

The psychodynamic play therapist is usually primarily non-directive in play sessions, following the lead of the client, who chooses toys and directs the play (Kottman, 2011). However, psychodynamic play therapy also has a more focused/directive component, where the therapist takes an active role by structuring sessions through the introduction of specific toys designed to facilitate clients reaching certain goals, activity playing with the child, and asking questions (Crenshaw, 2008; Mordock, 2015).

In psychodynamic play therapy, the primary goals are to help the client develop more mature defenses, re-adjust misperceptions and cognitive distortions, increase understanding of choices and consequences, explore fantasies and unrealistic desires, and strengthen ego functioning (Kottman, 2011; Mordock, 2015). The therapist's goal is to "explore, understand, and resolve the etiology of the arrests, fixations, regressions, defensive operations and so forth which bind up important sources of psychic energy to aid the resumption of normal development" (Lee, 2009: 43). The primary intervention strategies include interpretation, introducing structure, using specific toys to strengthen adaptive skills and help clients cultivate more mature defenses, asking questions, and (with children and adolescents) working with caretakers (Mordock, 2015).

The psychodynamic play therapy process moves through four stages of therapy (Mordock, 2015). The initial period involves establishing the working relationship, allaying anxiety, and defining the nature of play therapy. In the second stage, the therapist guides the child to explore underlying issues, deepen the relationship with the play therapist and become more engaged in the process of therapy. Often, the child works to master anxiety and conflicts. The third stage, establishing and implementing a formula for change, involves the therapist and the child moving into either talking about or playing through problematic situations. In this stage, the child often engages in repetitive play that helps him or her to deal with past traumatic situations and play out new solutions to problems. The play therapist offers a series of interpretations, and symptoms are discussed in different contexts. Termination is the fourth stage of the process—during this stage, the therapist helps the child work through the transition out of therapy.

The use of repetitive play in psychodynamic play therapy, as well as the encouragement of regressive play as a means of establishing state regulation, can find support in the neurosequential model. The therapist can use the strong relationship with the client to establish the safe environment necessary for the child to incorporate somatosensory integration and establish emotional regulation. The interpretations often used in psychodynamic play therapy can encourage cortical development of abstract thought patterns.

## Expressive arts therapies

"Creative arts therapies encourage clients to become active participants in the therapeutic process, and can energize the clients, redirect their attention and focus, and influence emotions" (Malchiodi, 2014: 4). According to Malchiodi (2014, 2015), creative and expressive arts therapies are important therapeutic approaches in the context of neuroscience and psychobiology because they emphasize (a) sensory-based interventions, (b) nonverbal communication, (c) right-hemisphere dominance, (d) emotional regulation, and (e) relational strategies. Art therapy, music therapy, dance/movement therapy, and drama therapy are usually considered the creative and expressive arts therapies. All of these approaches are predominantly directive/focused and can be used with children, adolescents, adults, and families, separately and combined with more directive/focused approaches to play therapy.

Art therapy is the intentional use of visual arts experiences and media to help clients gain insight into thoughts, emotions, bodily sensations, and behaviors (Graves-Alcorn and Green, 2014; Malchiodi, 2014, 2015). The art therapy process can provide clients with "(a) self-discovery, (b) personal fulfillment, (c) empowerment, (d) relaxation and stress relief, and (e) symptom relief and physical rehabilitation" (Graves-Alcorn and Green, 2014: 2). Although there are limited numbers of quantitative random, controlled experimental studies that support the efficacy of art therapy (Lombardi, 2014), there are several recent experimental studies that support the use of art therapy with sexually abused children (Pifalo, 2006), adolescent female offenders with low self-esteem (Hartz and Thick, 2005), and children on the autism spectrum (Epp, 2008).

Music therapy makes use of music to bring about positive changes in the psychological, social, cognitive, and/or physical functioning of children, adolescents, and adults (Malchiodi, 2014, 2015). Music therapists can use singing, musical improvising, songwriting, listening to and talking about music, and moving to music to help clients (Graves-Alcorn and Green, 2014; Hadley and Steel, 2014). In a 2004 meta-analysis of the effects of music therapy for children and adolescents with psychopathology, Gold, Voracek, and Wigram found that the effects of music therapy had a tendency to be greater for people who suffered from developmental and behavioral disorders than for people with emotional disorders.

Dance/movement therapy is the "psychotherapeutic use of movement to support integration of the mind, body, and spirit in the healing process" (Gray, 2015: 171). Dance and movement therapy is a combination of creative arts and somatic therapy, based on the belief that there is a connection between people's bodies and their thoughts, feelings, and behaviors (Levy, 2005). It is a directive, holistic approach that can be used with children, adolescents, and adults.

Drama therapy is an experiential method of using theatre techniques (e.g. storytelling, projective play, intentional improvisation, and performance) to effect change in the arenas of symptom relief, emotional and physical integration, and personal growth in children, adolescents, and adults (Irwin, 2014; Malchiodi, 2014, 2015). It can include interventions such as role-playing, theatre games, group dynamic activities, mime, puppetry, and improvisation (Graves-Alcorn and Green, 2014). Although the quantitative research into the efficacy of drama therapy is sparse, there are several promising outcome studies that tentatively support greater effectiveness of the treatment of traumatized clients when drama therapy is included (Haste and McKenna, 2010; McArdle *et al.*, 2011).

Expressive arts therapies can link naturally with the neurosequential model in using expressive arts as the canvas for the somatosensory and relational activities necessary for promoting social–emotional development. They can also facilitate emotional regulation and encourage abstract thought after these foundational experiences have occurred.

## Conclusion

Current directive and non-directive practices used with children, adolescents, and adults use a variety of creative means to connect with clients and help them to function better in their lives. Although not part of the initial development of the theories and therapeutic applications, the neurosequential model of brain development and its implications have been occurring within the therapeutic use of the interventions described in this chapter. For example, the importance of the relationship and its necessity to help the client move toward greater insight supported by the neurosequential model is also described in Adlerian, child-centred, and narrative play therapy theories as essential to the treatment process. Similarly expressive arts such as music, dance, and drama connect with different functions of the brain, helping the client to integrate sensory, cognitive, and emotional functioning. Overall, creative psychotherapies that include play and expressive arts optimize therapy results by incorporating concepts emphasized in the neurosequential model of brain development.

## References

Akay, S. (2013). *The effects of Adlerian play therapy on maladaptive perfectionism and anxiety in children*. Unpublished doctoral dissertation, University of North Texas, Denton.

Allan, J. (1997). Jungian play psychotherapy. In K. O'Connor and L.M. Braverman (eds) *Play Therapy Theory and Practice: A comprehensive presentation* (pp. 100–30). New York: Wiley.

Ammen, S. (2000). A play-based teen parenting program to facilitate parent/child attachment. In H. Kaduson and C. Schaefer (eds) *Short-Term Play Therapy for Children* (pp. 345–69). New York: Guilford.

Association for Play Therapy. (2014). *Play therapy defined*. Available at: www.a4pt.org/?page=PTMakesADifference (accessed 27 May 2016).

Axline, V. (1947). *Play Therapy: The inner dynamics of childhood*. Boston, MA: Houghton Mifflin.

Axline, V. (1964). *Dibs: In search of self*. New York: Ballantine Books.
Axline, V. (1969). *Play Therapy*. New York: Ballantine Books.
Barfield, S., Dobson, D., Gaskill, R., and Perry, B.D. (2012). Neurosequential model of therapeutics in a therapeutic preschool: Implications for work with children with complex neuropsychiatric problems. *International Journal of Play Therapy*, *21*(1), 30–44.
Blanco, P., Ray, D., and Holliman, R. (2012). Long-term child centered play therapy and academic achievement of children: A follow-up study. *International Journal of Play Therapy*, *21*(1), 1–13.
Booth, P., and Jernberg, A. (2010). *Theraplay: Helping parents and children build better relationships through attachment-based play* (3rd edn). San Francisco, CA: Jossey-Bass.
Booth, P., and Winstead, M. (2015). Theraplay: Repairing relationships, helping families heal. In D. Crenshaw and A. Stewart (eds) *Play Therapy: A comprehensive guide to theory and practice* (pp. 141–55). New York: Guilford.
Bratton, S.C., Ray, D., Rhine, T., and Jones, L. (2005). The efficacy of play therapy with children: A meta-analytic review of treatment outcomes. *Professional Psychology: Research & Practice*, *36*(4), 376–90.
British Association for Play Therapy. (2014). *Play therapy*. Available at: www.bapt.info (accessed 20 May 2016).
Carroll, F. (2009). Gestalt play therapy. In K.J. O'Connor and L.D. Braverman (eds), *Play Therapy: Theory and practice. Comparing theories and techniques* (2nd edn, pp. 283–315). Hoboken, NJ: John Wiley.
Cattanach, A. (2006). Narrative play therapy. In C. Schaeffer and H. Gerard Kaduson (eds) *Contemporary Play Therapy: Theory, research, and practice* (pp. 82–102). New York: Guilford.
Cattanach, A. (2008). *Narrative Approaches in Play with Children*. Philadelphia, PA: Jessica Kingsley.
Cavett, A. (2015). Cognitive-behavioral play therapy. In D. Crenshaw and A. Stewart (eds) *Play Therapy: A comprehensive guide to theory and practice* (pp. 83–98). New York: Guilford.
Crenshaw, D. (2008). *Therapeutic Engagement of Children and Adolescents: Play, symbol, drawing, and storytelling strategies*. Lanham, MD: Aronson.
Dillman Taylor, D., and Meany-Walen, K.K. (2015). Investigating the effectiveness of Adlerian play therapy with children with disruptive behaviors: A single-case research design. *Journal of Child & Adolescent Counseling*, *1*(2), 81–99.
Drewes, A., and Bratton, S. (2014). Play therapy. In E. Green and A. Drewes (eds) *Integrating Expressive Arts and Play Therapy with Children and Adolescents* (pp. 17–40). New York: Wiley.
Epp, K. (2008). Outcome-based evaluation of a social skills program using art therapy and group therapy for children on the autism spectrum. *Children & Schools*, *30*(1), 27–36.
Freud, A. (1946). *The Psychoanalytic Treatment of Children*. London: Imago.
Frey, D. (2015). Play therapy interventions with adults. In D. Crenshaw and A. Stewart (eds) *Play Therapy: A comprehensive guide to theory and practice* (pp. 452–64). New York: Guilford.
Gardner, B. (2015). Play therapy with adolescents. In D. Crenshaw and A. Stewart (eds) *Play therapy: A comprehensive guide to theory and practice* (pp. 439–51). New York: Guilford.

Garza, Y., and Bratton, S. (2005). School-based child-centered play therapy with Hispanic children: Outcomes and cultural considerations. *International Journal of Play Therapy*, *14*(1), 51–79.

Gaskill, R., and Perry, B. (2014). The neurobiological power of play. In C. Malchiodi and D. Crenshaw (eds) *Creative Arts and Play Therapy for Attachment Problems* (pp. 178–94). New York: Guilford.

Gold, C., Voracek, M., and Wigram, T. (2004). Effects of music therapy for children and adolescents with psychopathology: A meta-analysis. *Journal of Child Psychology & Psychiatry & Allied Disciplines*, *45*(6), 1054–63.

Graves-Alcorn, S., and Green, E. (2014). The expressive arts therapy continuum: History and theory. In E. Green and A. Drewes (eds) *Integrating Expressive Arts and Play Therapy with Children and Adolescents* (pp. 1–16). New York: Wiley.

Gray, A. (2015). Dance/movement therapy with refugee and survivor children. In C. Malchiodi (ed.) *Creative Interventions with Traumatized Children* (2nd edn, pp. 169–90). New York: Guilford.

Green, E. (2009). Jungian analytical play therapy. In K. O'Connor and L.M. Braverman (eds) *Play Therapy Theory and Practice: Comparing theories and techniques* (2nd edn, pp. 83–122). New York: Wiley.

Green, E. (2011). Jungian analytical play therapy. In C.E. Schaefer (ed.) *Foundations of Play Therapy* (2nd edn, pp. 61–86). Hoboken, NJ: Wiley.

Griffith, J., and Powers, R.L. (2007). *The Lexicon of Adlerian Psychology* (2nd edn). Port Townsend, WA: Adlerian Psychology Associates.

Guerney, L., and Guerney, B. (1987). Integrating child and family therapy. *Psychotherapy*, *24*(33), 609–14.

Hadley, S., and Steele, N. (2014). Music therapy. In E. Green and A. Drewes (eds) *Integrating Expressive Arts and Play Therapy with Children and Adolescents* (pp. 149–79). New York: Wiley.

Hartz, L., and Thick, L. (2005). Art therapy strategies to raise self-esteem in female juvenile offenders. *Art Therapy: Journal of the American Art Therapy Association*, *22*(2), 70–80.

Haste, E., and McKenna, P. (2010). Clinical effectiveness of drama therapy in the recovery from severe neuro-trauma. In P. Jones (ed.) *Drama as Therapy* (pp. 84–104). New York: Routledge.

Hoch, A. (2009). Trauma-focused cognitive behavioral therapy for children. In A. Rubin and D. Springer (eds) *Treatment of Traumatized Adults and Children* (pp. 179–253). Hoboken, NJ: Wiley.

Hug-Hellmuth, H. (1921). On the technique of child analysis. *International Journal of Psychoanalysis*, *2*, 287–305.

Irwin, E. (2014). Drama therapy. In E. Green and A. Drewes (eds) *Integrating Expressive Arts and Play Therapy with Children and Adolescents* (pp. 67–100). New York: Wiley.

Jafari, N., Mohammadi, M.R., Khanbani, M., Farid, S., and Chiti, P. (2011). Effect of play therapy on behavioral problems of maladjusted preschool children. *Iranian Journal of Psychiatry*, *6*(1), 37–42.

Jernberg, A. (1979). *Theraplay: A new treatment using structured play for problem children and their families*. San Francisco, CA: Jossey-Bass.

Klein, M. (1932). *The Psycho-analysis of Children*. London: Hogarth.

Knell, S. (1993). *Cognitive-Behavioral Play Therapy*. Northvale, NJ: Jason Aronson.

Knell, S. (2011). Cognitive-behavioral play therapy. In C.E. Schaefer (ed.) *Foundations of Play Therapy* (2nd edn, pp. 313–28). Hoboken, NJ: Wiley.

Knell, S., and Dasari, M. (2009). CBPT: Implementing and integrating CBPT into clinical practice. In A. Drewes (ed.) *Blending Play Therapy with Cognitive Behavioral Therapy* (pp. 321–52). Hoboken, NJ: Wiley.

Kottman, T. (2009). Adlerian play therapy. In K. O'Connor and L.M. Braverman (eds) *Play Therapy Theory and Practice: Comparing theories and techniques* (2nd edn, pp. 237–82). New York: Wiley.

Kottman, T. (2011). *Play Therapy: Basics and beyond* (2nd edn). Alexandria, VA: American Counseling Association.

Kottman, T., and Ashby, J. (2015). Adlerian play therapy. In D. Crenshaw and A. Stewart (eds) *Play Therapy: A comprehensive guide to theory and practice* (pp. 32–47). New York: Guilford.

Kottman, T., and Meany-Walen, K. (in press). *Partners in Play: An Adlerian approach to play therapy* (3rd edn). Alexandria, VA: American Counseling Association.

Lambert, S.F., LeBlanc, M., Mullen, J.A., Ray, D., Baggerly, J., White, J., and Kaplan, D. (2007). Learning more about those who play in session: The national play therapy in counseling practices project (phase 1). *Journal of Counseling & Development*, 85, 42–6.

Landreth, G. (2012). *Play Therapy: The art of the relationship* (3rd edn). New York: Routledge.

Landreth, G., and Bratton, S. (2006). *Child Parent Relationship Therapy (CPRT)*. New York: Routledge.

Lee, A. (2009). Psychoanalytic play therapy. In K. O'Connor and L.M. Braverman (eds) *Play Therapy Theory and Practice: Comparing theories and techniques* (2nd edn, pp. 25–82). New York: Wiley.

Levy, A. (2011). Psychoanalytic approaches to play therapy. In C. Schaefer (ed.), *Foundations of Play Therapy* (2nd edn, pp. 43–60). Hoboken, NJ: Wiley.

Levy, F. (2005). *Dance/Movement Therapy: A healing art*. Reston, VA: National Dance Association, American Alliance for Health, Physical Education, Recreation, and Dance.

Lew, A., and Bettner, B.L. (2000). *A Parent's Guide to Understanding and Motivating Children*. Newton Centre, MA: Connexions Press.

Lilly, J.P. (2015). Jungian analytical play therapy. In D. Crenshaw and A. Stewart (eds) *Play Therapy: A comprehensive guide to theory and practice* (pp. 48–65). New York: Guilford.

Lin, Y., and Bratton, S.C. (2015). A meta-analytic review of child-centered play therapy approaches. *Journal of Counseling & Development*, 93(1), 45–58.

Lombardi, R. (2014). Art therapy. In E. Green and A. Drewes (eds) *Integrating Expressive Arts and Play Therapy with Children and Adolescents* (pp. 41–66). New York: Wiley.

McArdle, P., Young, R., Quibell, T., Mosely, D., Johnson, R., and LeCouteur, A. (2011). Early intervention for at risk children: 3-year follow-up. *European Child & Adolescent Psychiatry*, 20(3), 111–20.

Malchiodi, C. (2014). Creative arts therapy approaches to attachment issues. In C. Malchiodi and D. Crenshaw (eds) *Creative Arts and Play Therapy for Attachment Problems* (pp. 3–18). New York: Guilford.

Malchiodi, C. (2015). Neurobiology, creative interventions, and childhood trauma. In C. Malchiodi (ed.) *Creative Interventions with Traumatized Children* (2nd edn, pp. 3–23). New York: Guilford.

Meany-Walen, K., Bratton, S., and Kottman, T. (2014). Effects of Adlerian play therapy on reducing students' disruptive behavior. *Journal of Counseling & Development, 92*, 47–56.

Meany-Walen, K.K., Bullis, Q., Kottman, T., and Dillman Taylor, D. (2015). Group Adlerian play therapy with children with off-task behavior. *Journal for Specialists in Group Work, 40*, 294–314.

Meany-Walen, K.K., Kottman, T., Bullis, Q., and Dillman Taylor, D. (in press). Adlerian play therapy with children with externalizing behaviors: Single case design. *Journal of Counseling & Development*.

Mills, J. (2015). StoryPlay: A narrative play therapy approach. In D. Crenshaw and A. Stewart (eds) *Play Therapy: A comprehensive guide to theory and practice* (pp. 171–85). New York: Guilford.

Mills, J., and Crowley, R. (2014). *Therapeutic Metaphors for the Child and the Child Within* (2nd edn). Philadelphia, PA: Brunner-Routledge.

Mordock, J. (2015). Psychodynamic play therapy. In D. Crenshaw and A. Stewart (eds) *Play Therapy: A comprehensive guide to theory and practice* (pp. 68–82). New York: Guilford.

Munns, E. (2011). Theraplay: Attachment-enhancing play therapy. In C.E. Schaeffer (ed.) *Foundations of Play Therapy* (2nd edn, pp. 275–96). Hoboken, NJ: Wiley.

Munns, E. (2014). Group Theraplay. In E. Prendiville and J. Howard (eds) *Play Therapy Today* (pp. 163–78). New York: Routledge.

Nash, J.B., and Schaefer, C. (2011). Play therapy: Basic concepts and practices. In C. Schaefer (ed.) *Foundations of Play Therapy* (2nd edn, pp. 3–13). Hoboken, NJ: John Wiley.

Oaklander, V. (1992). *Windows to Our Children: A Gestalt approach to children and adolescents*. New York: The Gestalt Journal Press. (Original work published 1978.)

Oaklander, V. (2006). *Hidden Treasure: A map to the child's inner self*. London: Karmac.

Oaklander, V. (2011). Gestalt play therapy. In C. Schaefer (ed.) *Foundations of Play Therapy* (2nd edn; pp. 171–86). Hoboken, NJ: Wiley.

Pifalo, T. (2006). Art therapy with sexually abused children and adolescents: Extended research study. *Art Therapy: Journal of the American Art Therapy Association, 23*(4), 181–5.

Ray, D. (2011). *Advanced Play Therapy: Essential conditions, knowledge, and skills for child practice*. New York: Routledge.

Ray, D., and Landreth, G. (2015). Child-centered play therapy. In D. Crenshaw and A. Stewart (eds) *Play Therapy: A comprehensive guide to theory and practice* (pp. 3–16). New York: Guilford.

Ryan, V., and Wilson, K. (2005). Adolescent play therapy from a nondirective stance. In L. Gallo-Lopez and C. Schaefer (eds) *Play Therapy with Adolescents* (pp. 96–120). Lanham, MD: Jason Aronson.

Schaefer, C., and Drewes, A. (eds) (2014). *The Therapeutic Powers of Play* (2nd edn). Hoboken, NJ: Wiley.

Schottelkorb, A.C., and Ray, D.C. (2009). ADHD symptom reduction in elementary students: A single-case effectiveness design. *Professional School Counseling, 13*(1), 11–22.

Siu, A. (2009) Theraplay in the Chinese World: An intervention program for Hong Kong children with internalizing problems. *International Journal of Play Therapy, 18*(1), 1–12.

Siu, A. (2014). Effectiveness of group play Theraplay on enhancing social skills among children with developmental disabilities. *International Journal of Play Therapy, 23*(4), 187–203.

Springer, C., and Misurell, J. (2012). Game-based cognitive-behavioral therapy individual model for child sexual abuse. *International Journal of Play Therapy, 21*(4), 188–201.

Sweeney, D., and Landreth, G. (2009). Child-centered play therapy. In K. O'Connor and L.M. Braverman (eds) *Play Therapy Theory and Practice: Comparing theories and techniques* (2nd edn, pp. 123–62). New York: Wiley.

Taylor de Faoite, A. (2011). The theory of narrative play therapy. In A. Taylor de Faoite (ed.) *Narrative Play Therapy: Theory & practice*. Philadelphia, PA: Jessica Kingsley.

VanFleet, R. (2003). Short-term filial therapy for families with chronic illness. In R. VanFleet and L.F. Guerney (eds) *Casebook of Filial Therapy* (pp. 65–83). Boiling Springs, PA: Play Therapy Press.

VanFleet, R. (2014). *Filial Therapy: Strengthening parent–child relationships through play* (3rd edn). Sarasota, FL: Professional Resource Press.

VanFleet, R., Ryan, S.D., and Smith, S. (2005). A critical review of filial therapy interventions. In L. Reddy and C.E. Schaefer (eds) *Empirically-Based Play Interventions for Children*. Washington, DC: American Psychological Association.

VanFleet, R., Sywulak, A., and Sniscak, C. (2010). *Child-Centered Play Therapy*. New York: Guilford.

Wettig, H., Coleman, A.R., and Geider, F.J. (2011). Evaluating the effectiveness of Theraplay in treating shy, socially withdrawn children. *International Journal of Play Therapy, 20*(1), 26–37.

Wettig, H., Franke, U., and Fjordbak, B. (2006). Evaluating the effectiveness of Theraplay. In C.E. Schaefer and H.G. Kaduson (eds) *Contemporary Play Therapy: Theory, research and practice* (pp. 103–235). New York: Guilford.

Wilson, K., and Ryan, V. (2005). *Play Therapy: A non-directive approach for children and adolescents* (2nd edn). London: Elsevier Science.

Yasenik, L., and Gardner, K. (2012). *Play Therapy Dimensions Model: A decision-making guide for integrative play therapists* (2nd edn). Philadelphia, PA: Jessica Kingsley.

Chapter 4

# Counseling skills in action with children, adolescents, and adults

*Lorri Yasenik and Ken Gardner*

Acquiring knowledge and skills in play and expressive art-based therapies is essential to psychotherapists who work with children, adolescents, and adults. Experiential activities in therapy assist the organization and capabilities of the developing and changing brain (Perry *et al.*, 1995, 2000; Schore, 1997). Clients across the lifespan often present in therapy with potentially chaotic, violent and/or cognitively and emotionally impoverished past experiences. Others come to therapy with transitional or developmental concerns. This chapter addresses the principles of play and creative therapies and the skills associated with working with these approaches from a neurodevelopmental point of view. The chapter will also address special considerations when one is examining the developing brain across three broad age bands, including children under 12, adolescents aged 13–18 years, and adults.

## Expressive and creative arts therapies: Practitioner skills and perspectives

The terms *expressive therapies* and *expressive arts therapies* are often used interchangeably with the term *creative arts therapies*. The term expressive arts therapies refers to a broad range of creative methods and experiential approaches that include, but are not limited to, all of the arts therapies and various forms of play therapy, including sand play, and they are based on the interrelatedness of the arts (Malchiodi, 2014; Richardson, 2015). In contrast, the term *creative arts therapies* is thought to specifically encompass art therapy, music therapy, drama therapy, dance/movement therapy, and poetry therapy (Malchiodi 2014).

A unifying reference point for expressive and creative arts therapies is that the underlying processes are experiential and action-oriented (Richardson, 2015). That is, all expressive arts therapies encourage the client to become an active participant, thereby energizing them, redirecting their attention and focus, and influencing their emotions. In this sense, creativity leads to the modification of behavior and is seen as a compilation of unconscious and/or conscious information channeled into some overt action (Graves-Alcorn and Green, 2014). However, the client's art is not simply viewed as an extension of his/her inner world: it also serves as a vehicle for communication and learning new ways of being in the world (Richardson, 2015). As in other forms of psychotherapy, the therapist acts as a guide and witness to the client's process of self-expression.

In the therapeutic setting, different modalities are sometimes purposefully combined, such as drawing, painting, music, or movement, as each offers opportunities for creative and symbolic self-expression. Emphasizing the value of self-selected expressive arts activities, Malchiodi (2005) argues that these activities facilitate a creative process of self-exploration that connects mind and body by stimulating all of the senses. Borrowing from current research in the cognitive neurosciences, it is clear that the self-creative process enhances right- and left-brain connections, necessary for healing, because it offers greater access to experiences, feelings and thoughts (Badenoch, 2008). Rubin (2005) further stresses that the awakening of a self-creative process in therapy serves as a protective factor, particularly for pre-adolescents, as it offers an internal structure for coping with future demands. Landgarten (1987) proposes that expressive media "can heighten or lower the client's affective state, influence freedom of self-expression, and circumvent defenses" (p. 7).

It is beyond the scope of this chapter to provide a comprehensive understanding of each form of creative or expressive therapy, as each functions as a distinct therapeutic intervention, with specific forms of education, training, and supervision requirements. Instead, this chapter will focus on the unifying therapeutic characteristics of play and art media, and the inherent power and/or healing properties of these in relation to symbolic expression. Play therapy and creative arts therapies make use of both verbal and nonverbal interactions and draw from a wide range of psychotherapy approaches, such as Humanistic, Psychodynamic, Gestalt, Adlerian, and Narrative (Malchiodi, 2008).

The expressive therapies continuum (ETC), originating with Kagin and Lusebrink (1978), is a conceptual model that provides direction for clinicians working in the various fields of expressive and creative arts psychotherapies to plan treatment based on integrated therapies. The continuum is an outgrowth of an earlier framework known as the *media dimension variables* (MDV; Graves, 1969). The earlier model was an attempt to define the use of art and expressive materials, therapeutically, as an exploitation of MDV (Graves-Alcorn and Green, 2014). Prior to this framework, art therapists primarily focused on projections from the unconscious, aided by the spontaneity of graphic or artistic expressions, and relatively little attention was given to the media with which these projections were promoted. Additionally, little consideration was given to the impact of providing directions to the client, or the degree of difficultly or complexity of the art project. Accordingly, Graves delineated three generalized media variables: (1) media properties, (2) structure, and (3) task.

The ETC was designed to be general enough to encompasses all basic modalities of expression, such as movement, sound, and words, by conceptualizing four stages of expression based on Piaget's developmental sequences (1962, 1969), representing four modes of interacting with the media (Kagin and Lusebrink,

1978). The sequence of expression follows Piaget's developmental sequence (1962, 1969) and, as will be discussed, has recently been placed into a neurosequential framework. The first stage, kinesthetic/sensory, recognizes the central role of sensorimotor play, as well as the use of related arts media, properties, structure or control, and level of complexity or cognitive understanding. In the kinesthetic/sensory level, the repetitive nature of sensory play by babies becomes embedded into a form of its own cognition (Graves-Alcorn and Green, 2014). The second level, the perceptual/affective level, occurs as actions or emotions begin to impact on feelings. Although the feelings do not yet have a verbal description, they begin to serve the function for which they were biologically intended, such as fear, which alerts us to danger. During the cognitive/symbolic level, form develops into signs, with meaning attached to the action that created the art form. As is noted by Kagin and Lusebrink (1978), the first three levels of ETC are similar to Bruner's theory of modes of representation: the enactive mode, which reflects past events through an appropriate motor response; the iconic mode, which organizes individual perceptions and images, selectively; and the symbolic mode, which is a system of designation and transformation of experience into a more abstract and complex way of representing internal and external reality (Bruner, 1964). The fourth level of the ETC is the creative level. This level is a synthesis of the other three levels, but is also distinct, owing to the integration, transformation, and expression of experiences into new forms.

Returning to an examination of media properties, it is apparent that the use of certain media may enhance or inhibit the process of development. For instance, a low-complexity/unstructured/fluid project, such as free-form finger-painting, provides a kinesthetic/sensory experience where the physical properties of the finger paints are primarily emphasized. If the child/client resonates with the fluidity of the paint on the wet paper, the experience should evoke a fluid, unrestricted response, as you might see in a 3-year-old engaged in finger-painting. That is, an unrestricted response would appear as the child/client playing joyfully; he/she may even develop a rhythm to create form. From a clinical standpoint, this same form of self-expression may be of considerable value to an adolescent or adult. However, as Graves-Alcorn and Green (2014) note, it is imperative that the clinician understands the media properties, knows how to introduce the media, and considers how to structure the therapy session.

Part of the creative arts therapist's role is to observe client responses, so as to better understand the client's reactions and enhance awareness of mind–body connections (Graves-Alcorn and Green, 2014). For instance, when working with fluid materials, such as finger paints, the child/client may describe the sensation as soft, gooey, or even yucky. Each of these sensations may be explored for additional background information or directed towards problem-solving or higher levels of awareness and insight, depending on the level of ETC that is operating.

Malchiodi (2012) has placed the ETC into a neurosequential framework as part of an intervention model called Trauma-Informed Expressive Arts Therapy. This model is based on the idea that expressive arts therapies help reconnect implicit (sensory) and explicit (declarative) memories of trauma, improve the client's capacity to self-regulate affect, and set the stage for integration and recovery (Malchiodi, 2014). The model has obvious applications to attachment work, as emphasis is placed on arts-based experiences that reinforce a sense of safety through self-soothing and positive attachment, while also building strengths through mastery experiences. As noted by Malchiodi (2014):

> In brief this means providing various opportunities for the individual to engage in creative experimentation that integrates experiences of unconditional appreciation, guidance, and support – experiences found in families with secure attachment relationships. In work with either a child or an adult, the goal is to help the individual recover the 'creative life' [Cattanach, 2008], and to regain a sense of well-being in oneself and in relationship to others.
>
> (p. 24–5)

Interventions at the Kinesthetic/sensory level that target the brainstem might include sensory use of materials, self-soothing experiences, such as music and movement activities, and rituals or structures in the presentation of materials. At this level, the targeted brain functions include stress responses, attachment/attunement to others, and ability to focus. Art activities at the kinesthetic/sensory level, which target the midbrain–diencephalon region, might include physically oriented activities such as crossing the midline, learning skills via art and play, and experiences of connection and approval. At this level, the targeted brain functions include motor skills, coordination, stress response, and attachment/attunement to others. Therapeutic activities targeting the limbic system, through working at the perceptual/affective level, might include interventions such as mask making, use of puppets for projective play and relational play, arts and crafts activities for creative expression, and skills enhancement. Targeted brain functions include affect regulation, relationships, and attachment/attunement. Finally, working at the cognitive/symbolic level, which addresses the cortex area of the brain, might include activities such as bibliotherapy, problem-solving activities, and arts for skill enhancement. As might be expected, sensory and affective-based methods may still be required at this level. Targeted brain functions include executive functions, self-image, social competence, and communication (Malchiodi, 2014).

As in other forms of psychotherapy, the therapist must consider issues such as the client's age, presenting issue, and stage of emotional and cognitive development in designing their interventions (Lombardi, 2014). During the initial assessment phase, the therapist primarily takes on the role of an observer, examining the client's verbal, nonverbal, visual, and metaphorical methods of communication (Rubin, 1999). Questions therapists might ask themselves include: What media did the client use or select, and what media did they decline? What was the nature of the client's engagement with the media—active/passive? Were there accompanying verbalizations, and, if so, what was the nature of these (i.e. directed towards the art media, the self, the therapist)? Were there noteworthy nonverbal gestures? How much time was spent undoing, reworking or erasing? Did the client cover up any images? Was a final product achieved? If so, what was the client's response? If not, what was the nature of the client's verbal/nonverbal responses?

Following the completion of a product, the therapist may engage in an inquiry by inviting the client to explore the product through open-ended questions that facilitate understanding or resonance with what they have created (Rubin, 2005). An inquiry can be undertaken with any form of symbolic expression, such as sand play, fantasy play, poetry, or movement. The inquiry typically begins with broad, open-ended questions, such as, "What can you tell me about this?" No attempt is made to immediately label or interpret any part of the drawing, activity, or product by bringing certain symbolic aspects of the image into conscious awareness. For example, if the image appears to be a tree, the therapist does not ask the client to tell them about the "tree," unless the client has already identified the object as a tree. Naming the object before the client names it runs the risk of the therapist assigning symbolic meaning to the image based on the therapist's personal associations or projections (Lombardi, 2014). As the inquiry continues, exploratory questions move from broad, open-ended questions towards more focused questions, as if moving down a funnel. The purpose is to assist the client in exploring all parts of the image, including borders and empty spaces. Once an image, activity or product has been named, the therapist might use this same label in their exploratory questions, but keep the inquiry directed at the symbolic level. For example, if the client has described an image as a tree, the therapist might inquire what the tree feels or senses in that environment, whether the tree is young or old, if there are other living things nearby the tree, whether the tree needs anything, if it feels safe, or, if the tree could speak, what might it say? Some questions invite specific projections, whereas others are relational in nature, inviting a broader phenomenological viewpoint or understanding of the client's world-view. At times, the client may signal a need for greater distance from talking in a direct or highly conscious manner, exemplified by the client who repeatedly states, "I don't know." Although this might be interpreted as a blocking response, the therapist should honor the client's need for distance, understanding that the client might be working from a lower level of conscious awareness and is not able to formulate an understanding of the symbolic image. In such a case, the therapist would return to broad, open-ended questions, moving towards the top of the funnel. When examined over the course of a session, the inquiry is tantamount to a weaving process, moving back and forth, from lower levels of conscious awareness to higher levels, based on the client's need for distance from the symbolic material and where they are at in the therapeutic process, including the therapeutic relationship (Yasenik and Gardner, 2014).

As the therapy process continues, the symbolic level of communication will inform the therapist as to the client's readiness or ability to work at a higher level of consciousness. At this point, prompts for engaging with the art media might become directive, such as, "Draw what anger looks like to you." Prompts might also become structuring, such as, "Draw a bridge that takes you from anger to calm."

Both the dimension of directiveness, represented through prompts or instructions that structure the task, and the dimension of consciousness, represented by the client's level of awareness of the symbolic nature of their communication, should be considered at any moment in therapy process. These two dimensions are represented in The Play Therapy Dimensions Model developed by the authors (Yasenik and Gardner, 2012). The model offers a decision-making guide for integrative play therapists, as well as those working in the expressive and creative arts therapies. To briefly illustrate this point, the intersection of the two primary dimensions, consciousness and directiveness, is reflected by a question such as, "Have you had moments when you were alone or abandoned, like the tree?" This question directs or focuses symbolic communication and is seen as falling on the directiveness side of the directiveness continuum. At the same time, the question invites a certain level of self-awareness, moving the client towards higher levels of conscious awareness along the consciousness dimension.

In discussing drama therapy approaches for children who have witnessed severe domestic violence, Weber (2005) notes that the making of *monster masks* provides a distanced (less conscious) method for children to explore their fears and begin to master them. However, with young children who lack the ego strength to wear the masks they make on their faces, their masks are made for stuffed animals to wear. To feel enough control and safety to explore the nature of these "monsters," structured (or directive) methods are used, such as only working on the masks for a short period of time and then placing them in a locked cabinet.

Therapists must also consider the influence of age and the stage of the client's development on the design of therapeutic activities. An older child might be encouraged to make two opposite masks, representing role and counter-role, where counter-role represents the victim and role represents the aggressor. Over time, the therapeutic focus with an older child might shift to the creation of a transformation mask, which takes on elements of strength and protection. In contrast, with a younger child, toy figures might initially be used to represent a fearful victim, rather than a mask, as masks may serve as too direct a trigger, being "under-distancing" for young children (Landy, 2001). To provide another layer of control, the toy figures might only be played with for a short period of time in the session, before being put away. For the young child, the transformation might be represented through thematic elements of pretend play, with various toys representing power or control, safety or reconnecting to others.

As noted by Irwin (2005), a central part of the drama therapist's work is the integration of spontaneous play and the dramatic structures of characters, plot, setting, and climax, to promote creativity and interpersonal growth. In her work with foster and adoptive children, Cattanach (2005) describes the blending of play and drama therapy through the use of a narrative approach. The use of narratives and stories assists children to make sense of their lives and learn empathy through imagining how characters in their story might feel. However, as Cattanach (2005) cautions, certain dominant stories the child holds about herself may not be helpful and can lead to victimization. Thus, the therapist might join the child in examining ways to shift or expand aspects of identity, through exploring certain roles and ways of being in the play. Cattanach (2005) emphasizes that working with stories and narratives in play is a collaborative process:

> In this kind of collaboration, the child can play with small toys and objects to create a dramatic event, draw a picture, or just make marks on clay or slime. But as they do, they tell a story about what they are doing. My role as therapist is to listen, perhaps ask questions about the story if required, and record the story by writing it down if the child requests it. If the play becomes a drama, then I might take a role if the child wishes. I might also share a story that might be congruent with the play of the child or as a way to deepen the relationship through the shared experience of telling and listening.
>
> (p. 233)

Regardless of the expressive or creative arts approach taken, one must use a developmental framework to guide decision-making. For instance, the growing cognitive capacities found in adolescence and the drive for values clarification can be accommodated through the design of drama/improvisation techniques that channel aspects of the adolescent's age-appropriate forms of rebelliousness. Emunah (2005) notes that, with this age group, "acting out" can be playfully channelled into "acting," fostering an opportunity for aggressiveness and rebelliousness, but within the safety and boundaries of a dramatic play that provides a window for self-observation.

We now turn to a more detailed understanding of how play and expressive arts therapists anchor their work to clients at different developmental stages.

## Special considerations when working with preschool children

Children of 3–6 years of age use play as a primary means to process their experiences and to consider alternative ways of viewing themselves and others. Play offers a vehicle for children to explore alternative ways to be in the world. Singer (1993) notes that preschoolers enter the symbolic play phase and, through this play, increase their understanding of construction of narrative, cause-and-effect thinking, and perspective taking. The development of play in children increases the exploration of reality as children move from egocentric and magical thinking to a more logical and reality-based view of the world.

Preschoolers demonstrate emerging language and communication skills, symbolic play ability, cognitive development (generalization and thinking in categories, increased memory, increased awareness of causality), increased self-regulation (ability to imagine and anticipate consequences of behavior), increased internalization of moral values and self-monitoring and an increased sense of self that grows out of competence and autonomy. In work with preschoolers, expressive and creative play-based activities are essential and are the primary form of communication. Play and expressive-based approaches are, therefore, the fundamental skill set necessary for practitioners working with this age band.

Both child development factors and the hierarchy of neurosequential development, as described by Perry (2006), are important to guiding interventions. The brain develops from the brainstem, which establishes state regulation to the midbrain, which incorporates somatosensory integration into the limbic brain development, which facilitates emotional regulation to cortical brain development, which relates to abstract thought. When considering materials and activities for work with young children, the therapist must consider the child's presentation, growing abilities, and developing brain. Available therapy materials need to correspond to the child's drive to continue to develop gross and fine motor skills, sensory awareness and need for experiences with objects that allow for exploration, sorting and aligning, building, movement and music, real-life symbols such as food and cooking items, and problem-solving objects. The materials to make available must therefore include such things as messy play items (sand, clay, water, finger paints, bubbles etc.), gross motor play items (balls, swords, scarves, pieces of fabric), colored blocks, real-life items (baby dolls, bottles, play food, plastic animals), puppets, stuffed toys, blankets, music, and objects that make sounds. Objects that replicate real-life experiences are important to children of 3–6 years. They are in the process of engaging in trial-and-error activities, as well as using fantasy to sort reality.

Preschoolers tend towards magical thinking, which is a way of interpreting reality through observing surface qualities versus using reasoning. Magical thinking "compromises accurate perceptions of reality" (Davies, 2004: 282). The preschooler's wishes, fantasies, and dreams may drive and influence their perceptions, as is seen through quick resolutions and magical endings in play scenarios and in day-to-day storytelling filled with both fantasy and the concrete reality of daily experiences. The reason puppets are so powerful for the preschooler relates to their belief in fantasy-based objects that move and act realistically (even if they do not look real) and their belief in things they cannot see (for example, the Easter bunny, Santa Claus or the tooth fairy). Children in this age group "assimilate magic with the concrete reality of everyday experience" as a type of weaving process (Davies, 2004: 284). Other cognitive processes for preschoolers include egocentric thinking, which affects the child's ability to assume another's perspective; attributing causes of events to the self; reversal of cause and effect; personalization; thinking in categories; and generalizations.

Young children have mental models of their interpersonal relationships, and these models shape how they view themselves and others. Fromberg (2002) has described social pretend play as partly driven by a child's internal schemas or internal working models (Bowlby, 1973). These schemas influence how children approach and negotiate their interactions with others during play, as indicated through various play scripts. Westen (1991) referred to affect tone as a dimension of interpersonal schemas that is indicative of a child's world-view. Children's affect tone can be measured in children's play through representations of relationships on a continuum of threatening/destructive/unsafe themes to safe/positive/supportive themes. Children may represent the world as being a good, safe, kind place or one that is bad, unsafe and harmful (Niec et al., 2009). If a child has been interrupted by incidental or ongoing trauma, the child's affect tone can be observed during play and expressive activities.

Preschoolers' emerging sense of self is related to a growing level of confidence and competence, autonomy, coping abilities, knowledge of sexual identity, and racial identity. Additionally, children aged 3–6 years are increasing their ability to categorize their experiences, which helps them to feel more in control and less vulnerable to anxiety. They are developing inner speech and private speech, which are used to sort experiences, rules and expectations. Four-to-six-year-olds are beginning to develop conscious inhibition of emotional expression and arousal (Davies, 2004). This level of consciousness allows the child to self-regulate, bringing their actions under control without as much external parental/caregiver support. When thinking about work with preschool children, the practitioner may reflect back to the ETC and be prepared to incorporate the first, kinesthetic/sensory level, which involves sensorimotor play using messy play materials, movement, sounds and other such media. Young children use all of their senses to make experiential meaning and to lay the foundation for perceptual/affective meanings, which are preverbal.

## Through the playroom window: Psychotherapy with 4-year-old Mathew

Mathew was referred to therapy to address a medical trauma. Mathew is from an intact family and is the older child of two; he has a younger infant sister. Mathew was scheduled for a serious dental surgical procedure and awoke out of the anaesthesia too early. He was described as in pain, hysterical, disoriented, and terrified at the time of awakening. After further medical attention and an attempt to manage his distress, he went home with his parents. Although distressed, he calmed down and reportedly played with some of his favorite toys later that day. The next morning, Mathew woke up and could not walk, apparently a rare but possible side effect of the anaesthesia. Mathew's parents were alarmed and rushed Mathew back to the hospital. His reaction to the hospital setting was significant, and he screamed and fought to leave the building. Mathew's paralysis was temporary (it lasted a full day), but distressing nonetheless. After this experience, Mathew reportedly was highly sensitive to sounds and being left alone in a room. He clung to his mother, was teary and had interrupted sleep, and he stopped playing with his favorite toys. He unfortunately had to return to the hospital setting for follow-up treatments. His parents were concerned that Mathew was regressing and that he was unable to emotionally process the medical procedure.

Upon reflection on the possible approaches to treatment for Mathew, the following factors were among those considered:

- Neurodevelopment: Mathew's midbrain and limbic areas of his brain were developing rapidly and normally. Generally, Mathew would be expected to be interested in large and fine motor skill activities, activities related to touch, movement, messy sensory play, finger-painting, objects that offered imaginative play opportunities, and dance. The medical trauma interruption reportedly affected Mathew's engagement in play, and he regressed to an earlier brainstem development need for being held, touched, and rocked by his mother. It would be expected that Mathew would need some similar basic movement and rhythm actions initially in therapy.
- Developmentally: Mathew would be expected to be drawn to play objects that would create opportunities to further his development of reality-testing and he would likely normally be using objects in a sensory and symbolic manner through pretend play, but, in his case, a need for more sensory play was hypothesized.
- Mathew appeared to have post-traumatic stress symptoms and likely needed to have some room to use materials that allowed for sensory integration such as sand, water, and various trays that offered different sensory experiences, such as rice and oatmeal. Mathew's play had been interrupted, and his experience of a predictable and safe world had been intruded upon. He would need play materials such as dolls, doctor's kit, flash light, food, blankets, and objects that also made noises.

Mathew entered the office with his mother and baby sister. He appeared frightened and was crying. He could not get past the entry without dropping to his knees and pulling his hoodie over his face. His mother, a highly sensitive parent, softly tried to soothe him. He would not let go of her hand and he was clearly distressed. After spending some time engaging with Mathew, I asked if he would like to come to the playroom with his mother. Mathew eventually agreed, and he and his mother and sister came to the playroom. Mathew kept his hoodie on and sat on the floor. I moved some objects closer to him, and he simply explored items by picking them up, moving them and then replacing them. He touched the sand and moved it around the tray. He did not move his body much during this session, and it appeared that the lights in the room bothered him.

The next session, Mathew quietly came into the office and waited with his mother. He agreed to come to the playroom with me without his mother. He was tentative and mostly nonverbal. I did not direct his play, and Mathew went to the sand and the water trays and moved the materials around with his hands. He picked up one of the baby dolls and immersed it in the sand and then the water. He picked up the baby lotion, squeezed some out and rubbed it all over the doll and then washed the baby off. The medical kit was close by, and Mathew used the items in it to check the baby's heart. He said, "the baby is sick and scared."

I used reflecting and tracking skills and noted that the "baby is afraid and does not feel well." Mathew agreed and handed me some items from the kit so that I could check the baby as well. I followed his lead and directions. I asked Mathew what the baby needed next. Mathew asked for band-aids and directed me to place band-aids all over the baby's face. The session ended with Mathew wrapping the baby up carefully and finding a safe place to put the baby until next time.

In the next few sessions, Mathew chose a number of airplanes that were named mommy, daddy, and baby planes. The planes were lined up and organized by size and powers. The baby planes had to stay back because they needed to be safe. Mathew directed me to take one of the planes, and I was to follow him. His plane quickly made an alarm sound, and he said to me to "fly" mine and "go quickly" in an alarmed tone, "because there is a fire!" I followed his lead, and we flew the planes over to where the baby dolls were and shot pretend water on the babies and flew back to other "little planes." The big planes then reported to the little planes that everything was ok and it was a close call but the fire was out. This type of repetitive, alarmed, emergency-oriented pretend play that focused on the need to act quickly and put out fires with limited time to respond all appeared to be what Mathew needed to do to feel back in control in his life and was in part a psychological/emotional repair. Mathew demonstrated the use of reality-oriented objects (dolls, doctor's kit, idea of time and the clock) and fantasy play (planes flying and putting out pretend fires) in order to demonstrate his need for control. Mathew continued this type of gross movement play using his whole body (and requiring me to do the same) until there was a lessening of the urgency and he claimed that there were no further emergencies. Mathew's parents reported improvement at home and that he had no negative reaction to his last medical check-up. Through sensory play, gross motor and fantasy pretend play, Mathew recovered and made sense of the intrusive medical trauma. Through play, Mathew's world-view shifted from an unsafe, scary place where unpredictable emergencies occurred to a safe, organized, protective place.

## Special considerations when working with children in middle childhood

Middle childhood spans from about 6 years of age to the onset of puberty at 11–12 years. During middle childhood, children thematically focus on increasing skills and learning how to do things. There is a transitional phase between early childhood and middle childhood where skills and abilities are somewhat inconsistently present. Cross-culturally, there is some evidence that children between 5 and 8 years old are more capable of reasoning, learning, and perceiving reality accurately (Davies, 2004). Rogoff (1998) points out that, in most cultures, children begin a formal education or apprenticeship when they are 5–6 years old. Middle school-aged children gradually increase the accuracy of their perception of reality. Egocentrism is steadily replaced by decentration, which allows children to distinguish between subjective and objective reality. In middle childhood, magical thinking declines and is replaced by cause-and-effect thinking and the increased use of logic and reasoning. By the age of 7, children have a relatively well-developed understanding of spatial organization, time orientation, distinctions between parts and wholes, seriation, and auditory processing. Children's memories improve because they are better able to register and categorize things, as well as being able to sustain their attention more (Davies, 2004).

Those in middle childhood can now use their logical thinking and representational competence to delay impulsive behavior so that they can stay focused on the attainment of goals. Children in this stage of development have internalized values, expectations, rules and social norms, as well as better-developed defense mechanisms, which all contribute to higher levels of self-regulation. As cognitive development continues, the child's play activities and use of fantasy also move forward. When working clinically with children in middle childhood, the practitioner will notice that 6–7-year-olds (and older) will tend to demonstrate physical skills and intellectual competence through play activities and check to see they have an audience to witness their actions. Children of this age are likely to use play materials to challenge themselves to more complex levels of a game, making up new rules and strategies as they go, for instance. Children who are 7 years and older have an increased ability to narrate their play and can tell an organized story during fantasy or projective play. Expressive activities are now laden with meaning-making by the child. The older the child (beyond 7 years old), the more likely she/he can define space and the relative size of objects/figures. Case (1998) notes that, by age 10, children's drawings reflect lines that demonstrate spatial and linear perspectives and more consistently represent what the eye sees. Case also points out that, after the age of 7, children incorporate that numbers represent sequences and they begin to understand how time is organized. Time begins to take on new meaning in projective play. Additionally, during fantasy play, 8–10-year-olds make use of wordplay, jokes, and metaphors, and their play actions include displacement of feelings, wishes and concerns into imaginary scenarios. Expressive activities are more organized, realistic, and multilayered.

A practitioner will likely observe a child in middle-to-late childhood including things in their play that relate beyond the immediate family, as they are more inclusive of peers and establishing their role with others; they also have a greater focus on community, as this is a period of rapid social development. Of importance here is the knowledge that children begin to think beyond the self and recognize the needs of others (Eisenberg and Fabes, 1998). They are highly attuned to adult standards and they (particularly in public) try to follow those rules. This stage of development falls into what Kohlberg (1984) describes as the authority and social-order orientation of moral development.

Working with middle school-aged children requires more projective materials related to art (paint, drawing materials, clay) and play (miniatures, drama, masks, games). Returning to the ETC, children in this age group are often working at the perceptive/affective level (actions begin to impact feelings) and the cognitive/

symbolic level (form develops into signs, with meaning attached to the action that created the form).

## Through the playroom window: Psychotherapy with 11-year-old Mark

Mark was referred to private counseling by his school counselor. Mark had reportedly talked to the school counselor about feeling highly stressed and at times picked on or bullied by other children at school (one boy in particular). Mark's parents reported that he was highly sensitive and cried easily. Mark, at times when he was upset over something or if he felt badly for a friend, would not just become teary, but would cry for a long period of time and not be able to soothe himself. The following bullet points indicate information gathered during intake meetings:

- referral by school counselor in March;
- intact family—both parents attend intake;
- mother defers entirely to father;
- father presented as anxious, on edge of chair—appeared very sensitive;
- difficulties reported by parents begin with Mark being bullied at school but are noted as mostly resolved (but Mark does not generally differentiate teasing from insults);
- "incident" that occurred right after Christmas—sister said "I had a very bad dream that Mark is going to die";
- Mark shared that what his sister reported was not a dream, and his sister noted she saw Mark put a knife to his throat one day and she was afraid—parents want to know is "everything ok now?"

Upon reflection on the possible approaches to treatment for Mark, the following factors were among those considered:

- Neurodevelopment: Mark's midbrain, limbic and cortical areas of his brain were normally developing. Generally, Mark would be expected to be interested in activities related to ritualized games with rules and the use of fantasy play as a form of displacement of feelings and wishes into imaginary scenarios. Mark was viewed as highly emotionally reactive with a low sensory threshold. His arousal states were on high alert, not owing to trauma, but rather owing to temperament. With the limbic system highly "online," he experienced an interruption in accessing abstract and concrete thinking and problem-solving.
- Developmentally: Mark would be expected to be drawn to play materials that offered ways to express competence and a mounting sense of confidence. Complex themes related to projective play objects and the ability to narrate realistic themes and scenarios would be predicted.

- Mark's high sensitivity and limited ability to emotionally self-regulate interrupted his cognitive skills (cortical area of brain) in meaning-making, management of feeling states, and problem-solving. Although Mark was highly verbal and presented with some abstract reasoning and concrete thinking, other adults in his world had not been able to assist him to self-regulate through the use of cognitive verbal processing. Mark needed some projective materials on to which to displace his feelings, providing him with distance and an opportunity to externalize his worries and concerns.

Mark initially attended the introductory part of the session with his father. He presented as highly verbal, earnest, and highly motivated to "feel better." He seemed to have some awareness of his sensitivity to other people's emotions and confirmed that he felt easily sad and, when he perceived others as being hurt or harmed, would cry for long periods of time. He noted he cried at home and at school. He also reported that the bullying his father had talked about had subsided and, upon hearing more about it, the actions of the boy who was described as a "bully" extended to other kids in his class as well. The "incident" of previously picking up a knife and putting it to his throat was also put forward. Mark was unsure why he had felt so bad that day. His actions, feelings, and words had not come together for him. His father remained anxious and worried for Mark.

Mark's verbal presentation may lure many talk therapists into doing cognitive therapy with him. What was noticed, however, was that Mark's awareness had limitations, and his distress continued after having talked to a school counselor and to his parents about his feelings. Mark's temperament also suggested that his sensory system was easily overloaded, and, when this occurred, he was unable to use age-appropriate coping and problem-solving skills; Mark had little to no filter and he let most emotional matters in and then could not process how he felt. During the first session, Mark was offered materials that would assist him to externalize his need for a better filter. Although many therapists might have tried to talk to Mark about his need for more self-protection, it appeared that what would be more helpful was if Mark could make use of objects and move them around. This way, he might be able to create a symbolic representation of protection.

Mark was invited to use the sandtray and miniatures and was asked to pick an object that could be him. A metaphor was presented to Mark in the following way: "Mark, I noticed that you have a very kind and sensitive heart. I think sometimes it is easy for others to attack your heart and then you feel sad and upset. I think your heart needs more protection, like an invisible shield." Mark agreed with the metaphor by nodding his head. He chose an object to be him and placed it in the middle of the sandtray. The next instruction was to find some objects that could be used to create a shield or line of protection all around him (the figure). Mark chose a number of jewels and shiny stones to create layers of protection around the figure. He then used clay to create a protective cover for the figure, where the figure could see out but "no one could see in." This externalizing activity helps the child to work at the cognitive/symbolic level. It also helps provide the child with a way to see the self and make use of symbols to build on abstract notions of strength and emotional boundaries. Words can be added to the symbols chosen.

Mark worked with the sandtray and miniatures over five sessions. His ability to put words to feelings and to identify ways to avoid "heart attacks" evolved. He placed objects into the scenes that were the "attackers" and then used play actions and objects to ward the attackers off. He asked if I could take action pictures of him hitting the attackers with a catapult, which I did (see Figure 4.1).

Near the end of the process for Mark, he reported that he knew why he had been so upset and had thought of using a knife to harm himself. He noted that his father was always so worried and asked him so many questions and he felt he could not say anything to stop him. I asked him if he could draw a picture for his father to show him how he felt, and Mark immediately agreed. During a session with his father Mark directly practiced setting more emotional boundaries with his father through his drawing and accompanying words. Mark's father was very receptive to him, and Mark began to use his words as a shield for his heart. This approach to psychotherapy fit Mark's age and stage of development in that he needed to access his emerging cognitive and emotional skills, but through being provided with some symbols, distance, and a meaningful metaphor.

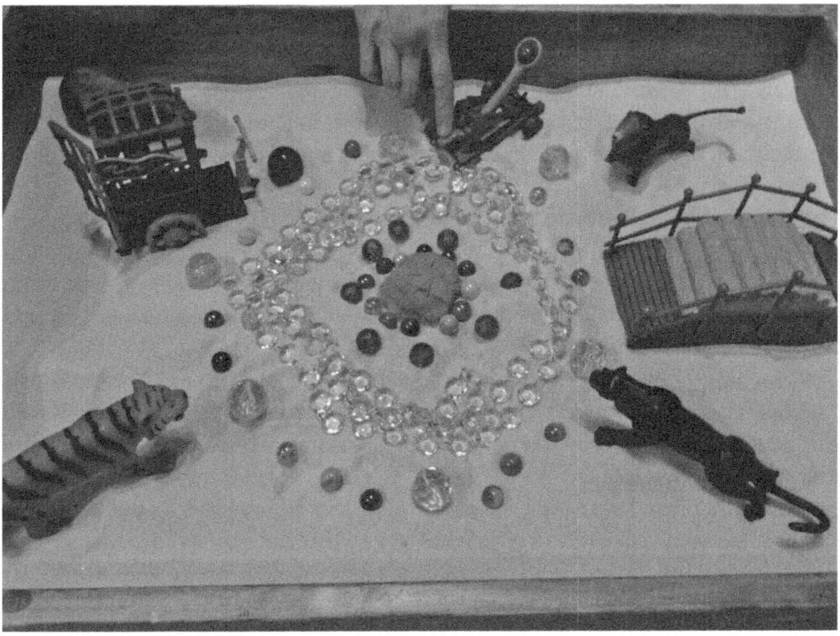

*Figure 4.1* Mark and the catapult

## Special considerations when working with adolescents and adults

Adolescence is considered to begin around age 12 and lasts until age 20 plus. Neurodevelopmentally, the brain continues to change, as has been demonstrated by brain scans of children over time. There is evidence that, over the course of childhood, the volume of gray matter (thin folding outer layer) in the cortex increases and then declines. The highest volume of gray matter can be measured during early adolescence. This suggests that the maturation of the brain does not taper and end until the early 20s. It would appear that different parts of the cortex develop at different rates, with areas involving basic functions (sensory processing and movement) maturing first, and the control of impulses and planning ahead maturing last. An understanding of region-specific changes in cortical development is necessary when comparing the processing capacities of adolescents with those of adults. In adolescence, the part of the brain that is related to emotional processing is fully online and maybe more so than in adults, but the emotional impulsive response is still maturing. This increases the draw towards novelty and risk-taking without thought for consequences.

Accompanying the cognitive-developmental changes in adolescence, most notably the ability to think abstractly, are dramatic changes in the self-structure across the substages of adolescence (Harter, 1999). In early adolescence, abstractions about the self are based on a new-found cognitive ability to integrate trait labels into higher-order self-concepts. In turn, these self-concepts enhance self-/other acceptance as social attributes are emphasized, as well as self-representations that focus on competencies, such as intellectual abilities and positive affects (e.g. "I'm cheerful"). Moving from the early to middle and later stages of adolescence, there is a proliferation of "selves" that vary as a function of social context. For example, there is movement from self with father and mother to self with close friends, romantic partners, as well as self in the role of student or athlete. Harter (1999) therefore argues that a critical developmental task during the substages of adolescence is the construction of multiple selves that vary across different roles and relationships. Cognitive-developmental advances not only permit increasing degrees of differentiation, but collaborate with socialization pressures to develop different selves in relational contexts (Erikson, 1968).

Rosenburg (1986) identifies another component of the differentiation process, noting that, as one moves through adolescence, one is more likely to be treated differently according to the relational contexts. Harter's research (1999) supports this trend: the overlap in self-attributes generated for different social contexts ranges from 25 to 30 percent among seventh and eighth graders and decreases during adolescence to a low of approximately 10 percent among older adolescents.

Erikson's (1950) theory of psychosocial development views adolescence as spanning the ages of 12–19, with a transition into adulthood. The stage of identity versus role confusion is viewed as a major stage that includes integrating multiple roles as an adult, increased independence and increased identity formation, particularly the sexual and occupational identities. Bee (1992) notes that, at the end of this stage, a reintegration of sense of self occurs where the adolescent's body image also changes. Successful transition from this stage leads to fidelity, meaning that the adolescent commits to his-/herself and forms an acceptance of others, even if differences are apparent.

## Through the therapy room window: Psychotherapy with a 15-year-old

Lisette was a referred to therapy by her parents. At the time of the referral, Lisette was also attending the Eating Disorder Clinic Day Program. Lisette's parents decided that she needed more one-on-one counseling, and she was not able to get this at the clinic, and they were further concerned she was not progressing. Just before the referral, Lisette's heart rate and other vitals had reached an all-time low, and she had been hospitalized. She was also considered significantly underweight.

Lisette reported no history of abuse. Her parents were supportive but felt weary and hopeless about their daughter's situation. They attended any group or family session requested of them at the clinic. Lisette apparently decided to go on a diet after spending a summer with her teenage cousin two years previously. Her cousin taught her about how to control what and when she ate. Six months later, Lisette was diagnosed with anorexia nervosa. Lisette was described as highly attention-seeking and a hypochondriac. Prior to the diagnosis of anorexia, Lisette would often make up various serious symptoms in an attempt to prove to her parents she had a life-threatening disease. Her parents were convinced that she felt she had succeeded in gaining their full attention. Lisette appeared mostly satisfied with her situation and saw no reason to do anything different, because she did not want to get fat. Although Lisette put on a good front, she was now trapped in her disorder. She craved various fun foods and become obsessed with the food channel and baking. She gained some satisfaction watching others eat. Lisette claimed to be afraid of many things and was nervous not having both parents home at the same time. She had also decided she was too afraid to learn how to drive. When she was ill from loss of weight, she stopped being able to attend school.

Upon reflection on the possible approaches to treatment for Lisette, the following factors were among those considered:

- Neurodevelopment: Lisette's midbrain, limbic and cortical areas of her brain were normally developing. Generally, Lisette's development would include an increase in abstract reasoning to solve problems and an increase in complex cognitive processing. Lisette appeared to be processing in a less advanced way than others at her age and stage of development. The limbic system appeared to be "lit," and she seemed to need some assistance with emotion regulation in order to identify the risks she was now taking with her life.
- Developmentally: Lisette would be expected to be drawn to materials that offered symbolic and abstract meaning. Complex themes related to self, peers

and social order would likely be observable. Lisette would likely be able to put words to feeling states when she was feeling calm. Lisette should be in the identity formation stage of development. It would appear at the onset of therapy that Lisette was not easily embracing her independence phase and she was needing, instead, a sense of being cared for and attended to; a dependency was noted. Although Lisette's parents were highly supportive, she struggled with accepting their attempts.

Based on Lisette's age and stage of development, it was important to begin to work with her emerging sense of independence and identity formation. Lisette was capable of making use of symbols in more abstract ways than the children discussed in the previous two age groups. She could now think about thinking about herself. It appeared that Lisette needed to work with the parts of herself, and so the following instruction was provided: Using any of the miniatures on the shelf, make a scene of the parts of you. Think of things that make you unique or things that are important to you. Lisette chose a number of miniatures and placed them in the sandtray. Beginning with Lisette's view of self began to mark the path towards facilitating her to have a relationship with herself. Through objects, Lisette illuminated the following disconnected parts of self: a ninja that represented the irritated part of her and the part that was most irritated with her mother; a blue dog that represented a sad and blue part of her; a pig that represented how she saw herself, "with a pot belly"; a helicopter with a guy inside that represented "a hidden real self"; an army tank that represented the war with her parents over food and eating; a puppy that represented her desire to be a veterinarian in the future; a girl in a hospital bed who represented the sick part of her; trees that represented how much she liked the outdoors; a cartoon character who represented her worries and what she named as her insecurities; and the horned guy who represented her anorexia, and she stated, "he is mean and big and hard to get rid of and he has a lot of power."

Through symbolizing parts of self, Lisette began an expressive and direct dialogue. This beginning activity provided a window into some of her hopes for the future, fears, self-image, and relational issues. This information provided a path towards working with her to strengthen her internally to deal with the anorexia and also offered a way to externalize the anorexia so that it could be approached with less defensiveness. From this beginning, Lisette was asked to work with a number of parts of self through sand play. She did a number of trays that followed each other. They had titles such as "The internal war," "Gaining protection from the big guy," "Peace," "Friends and family," to name a few. Lisette worked each session with a new title provided by the author, and she began to work more deeply with her "self." Identity issues and body image issues emerged, as well as her fear of growing up. Over time, the symbols were used to speak to one another, and an internal dialogue was possible. Later in the process, Lisette's parents were part of a sand play session. Lisette was able to speak to them about her fears and her needs. They gained insight into their daughter's worry about not being special or central to them. The process was deepened by the parents' choosing symbols to speak to Lisette's symbols.

Over time, the grip of the eating disorder lessened. Lisette stopped attending the day clinic and also began to gain weight. She also began to allow herself some fun foods again. The overall life-threatening issues diminished, and Lisette returned to school. Lisette appeared to move more fully into the identity formation phase of development.

## Key points

- This chapter has provided an overview of the perspectives, skills, and techniques used by play and expressive art-based therapists.
- Principles and skills associated with working from a neurodevelopmental framework are highlighted, along with special considerations for the application of directive and non-directive techniques.
- When working with expressive media, the therapist must carefully track movement along the dimension of consciousness and be prepared to remain working at the symbolic/unconscious level, so as not to activate defenses or overpower the client's ego resources.
- Engagement of the creative process in therapy, through various forms of self-expression, taps into the healing properties of symbolic expression and enhances right- and left-brain connections.
- The ETC model offers therapists a conceptual tool for planning treatment based on an integrative, neruosequential framework.
- A primary role of the creative psychotherapist is to observe the client's response to different media and facilitate the client's exploration of their creation through a recursive inquiry process.
- Regardless of the specific expressive approach taken, the therapist should use a developmental framework to guide decision-making. Accordingly, three developmental stages are highlighted, with accompanying case studies examined through the play/therapy room window.
- Play offers a way for preschool children to explore alternative ways to be in the world. The development of play increases the child's exploration of reality, moving from egocentric and magical thinking to a more logical and reality-based view of the world. The case of 4-year-old Mathew highlights the need to conceptualize the referral issue on multiple levels: developmentally, neurodevelopmentally (midbrain and limbic areas), and based on post-traumatic stress symptoms.
- There is a transitional phase from early to middle childhood where skills and abilities are somewhat inconsistently present. Middle-school children increase in their accuracy of perception of reality, and egocentrism is replaced by decentration. The case of 11-year-old Mark highlights the manner in which high levels of sensitivity and limited abilities to emotionally self-regulate

interrupted his cognitive skills (cortical area of the brain) in meaning-making, management of feeling states, and problem-solving. The presentation of a metaphor, as part of an externalizaton strategy, provided Mark with the opportunity to work at the cognitive/symbolic level and a way to see the self and build on abstract notions of strength and emotional boundaries.
- A critical developmental task during the substages of adolescence is the construction of multiple selves that vary across different roles and relationships. Lisette, a 15-year-old struggling with an eating disorder, was asked to work with a number of parts of self through sand play. This case illustrates movement, more fully, into the identity-formation phase of development.
- Overall, by emphasizing neurosequential and developmental research, the therapist is equipped to conceptualize the referral concerns and develop appropriate expressive therapies tailored to the holistic needs of the client.

## References

Balendoch, B. (2008). *Being a Brain-wise Therapist*. New York: Norton.
Bee, H.L. (1992). *The Developing Child*. London: HarperCollins.
Bowlby, J. (1973). *Attachment and Loss: Vol. 2. Separation*. New York: Basic Books.
Bruner, J.S. (1964). The course of cognitive growth. *American Psychologist*, *19*, 1–15.
Case, R. (1998). The development of conceptual structures. In W. Damon, D. Kuhn and R.S. Siegler (eds) *Handbook of Child Psychology: Vol. 2. Cognition, perception, and language* (5th edn, pp. 745–800). New York: Wiley.
Cattanach, A. (2005). Co-working with adoptive parents to support family attachments. In A.M. Weber and C. Haen (eds) *Clinical Applications of Drama Therapy in Child and Adolescent Treatment* (pp. 227–44). New York: Brunner-Routledge.
Cattanach, A. (2008). *Play Therapy with Abused Children* (2nd edn). London: Kingsley.
Davies, D. (2004). *Child Development: A practitioner's guide*. New York: Guilford Press.
Eisenberg, N., and Fabes, R.A. (1998). Prosocial development. In W. Damon and N. Eisenberg (eds) *Handbook of Child Psychology. Vol. 3. Social, emotional and personality development* (5th edn, pp. 701–78). New York: Wiley.
Emunah, R. (2005). Drama therapy and adolescent resistance. In A.M. Weber and C. Haen (eds) *Clinical Applications of Drama Therapy in Child and Adolescent Treatment* (pp. 107–20). New York: Brunner-Routledge.
Erikson, E.H. (1950). *Childhood and Society*. New York: Norton.
Erikson, E.H. (1968). *Identity, Youth and Crisis*. New York: Norton.
Fromberg, D.P. (2002). *Play and Meaning in Early Childhood Education*. Boston, MA: Allyn & Bacon.
Graves, S. (1969). Media dimension variables in art therapy. *Congress of the American Society of Psychopathology of Expression*, Boston, MA.
Graves-Alcorn, S.L., and Green, E.J. (2014). The expressive arts therapy continuum: History and theory. In E.J. Green and A. Drewes (eds) *Integrating Expressive Arts and Play Therapy with Children and Adolescents* (pp. 1–16). Hoboken, NJ: John Wiley.

Harter, S.H. (1999). *The Construction of the Self: A developmental perspective*. New York: Guilford Press.
Irwin, E.C. (2005). Facilitating play with non-players: A developmental perspective. In A.M. Weber and C. Haen (eds) *Clinical Applications of Drama Therapy in Child and Adolescent Treatment* (pp. 3–24). New York: Brunner-Routledge.
Kagin, S.L., and Lusebrink, V.B. (1978). The expressive therapies continuum. *Art Psychotherapy*, 5(4), 171–80.
Kohlberg, L. (1984). *Essays on Moral Development: Vol. 2. The psychology of moral development*. New York: Harper & Row.
Landgarten, H. (1987). *Family Art Psychotherapy: A clinical guide and casebook*. New York: Bruner/Mazel.
Landy, R. (2001). *New Essays in Drama Therapy: Unfinished business*. Springfield, IL: Charles C. Thomas.
Lombardi, R. (2014). Art therapy. In E. Green and A. Drewes (eds) *Integrating Expressive Arts and Play Therapy* (pp. 41–66). Hoboken, NJ: Wiley.
Malchiodi, C.A. (2005). *Expressive Therapies*. New York: Guilford Press.
Malchiodi, C.S. (2008). *Creative Interventions for Traumatized Children*. New York: Guilford Press.
Malchiodi, C.A. (2012). Art therapy and the brain. In C.A. Malchiodi (ed.) *Handbook of Art Therapy* (2nd edn, pp. 17–26). New York: Guilford Press.
Malchiodi, C.S. (2014). Creative arts therapy approaches to attachment issues. In C.S. Malchiodi and D.A. Crenshaw (eds) *Creative Arts and Play Therapy for Attachment Problems* (pp. 36–95). New York: Guilford Press.
Niec, L.N., Yopp, J., and Russ, S.W. (2009). *Validity of the interpersonal themes in playscale*. Unpublished manuscript, Department of Psychology, Central Michigan University, Mt. Pleasant, MI.
Perry, B.D. (2006). Applying principles of neurodevelopment to clinical work with maltreated and traumatized children. In N.B. Webb (ed.) *Working with Traumatized Youth in Child Welfare* (pp. 27–52). New York: Guilford Press.
Perry, B.D., Hogan, L., and Marlin, S.J. (2000). Curiosity, pleasure and play: A neurodevelopmental perspective. *Haaeyc Advocate*, 9–12.
Perry, B.D., Pollard, R., Blakely, T., Baker, W., and Vigilante, D. (1995). Childhood trauma, the neurobiology of adaptation and 'use-dependent' development of the brain: How 'states' become 'traits'. *Infant Mental Health Journal*, 16(4), 271–91.
Piaget, J. (1962). *Play, Dreams and Imitation in Childhood*. New York: W.W. Norton.
Piaget, J. (1969). *The Child's Conception of Time*. New York: Routledge Kegan Paul.
Richardson, C. (2015). *Expressive Arts Therapy for Traumatized Children: A four-phase model*. New York: Routledge.
Rogoff, B. (1998). Cognition as a collaborative process. In W. Daman, D. Kuhn and R.S. Siegler (eds) *Handbook of Child Psychology, Vol. 2, Cognition, perception, and language* (5th edn, pp. 745–800). New York: Wiley.
Rosenburg, M. (1986). Self-concept from middle childhood through adolescence. In J. Suls and A.G. Greenwald (eds) *Psychological Perspective on the Self* (vol. 3, pp. 107–35). Hillside, NJ: Erlbaum.
Rubin, J.A. (1999). *Introduction to Art Therapy: Sources and resources*. New York: Routledge.
Rubin, J.A. (2005). Child Art Therapy (25th Anniversary edn). Hoboken, NJ: Wiley.

Schore, R. (1997). Rethinking the brain: New insights into early development. Summary from conference: Brain development in young children: New frontiers for research, policy and practice. Families and Work Institute: New York.

Singer, J.L. (1993). Imaginative play and adaptive development. In J.H. Goldstein (ed.) *Toys, Play and Child Development* (pp. 6–26). Cambridge, UK: Cambridge University Press.

Weber, A.M. (2005). 'Don't hurt my mommy'. Drama therapy for children who have witnessed severe domestic violence. In A.M. Weber and C. Haen (eds) *Clinical Applications of Drama Therapy in Child and Adolescent Treatment* (pp. 25–44). New York: Brunner-Routledge.

Westen, D. (1991). Social cognition and object relations. *Psychological Bulletin, 109*, 429–55.

Yasenik, L., and Gardner, K. (2012). *Play Therapy Dimensions Model: A decision-making guide for integrative play therapists*. London: Jessica Kingsley.

Yasenik, L., and Gardner, K. (2014). The consciousness dimension in play therapy: Sharpening the play therapist's focus and skills. In E. Prendiville and J. Howard (eds) *Play Therapy Today: Contemporary practice with individuals, groups and carers* (pp. 29–46). New York: Routledge.

Part II

# Working with the brainstem and midbrain

Part I provided an introduction to conceptualizing play and expressive arts therapies on a neurodevelopmental continuum in order to provide developmentally appropriate and sequential interventions for child, adolescent and adult clients. Beginning with understanding the importance of creating a sense of safety, both physically and emotionally, a calm state enables the social engagement system to function. Principles of the polyvagal theory were presented, enabling the therapist to further understand the nature of the stress response and its relevance to the facilitation of both self-regulation and co-regulation. The matching of treatment approaches to physiological and developmental needs and the neurobiological sequelae of trauma provides a new lens through which the selection of specific play therapy modalities can be understood. An overview was presented of directive and non-directive approaches, ranging from somatosensory through to creative and symbolic play, which can help organize the respective parts of the brain. In Part II, modalities that address the brainstem and midbrain, the areas necessary for the experience, processing and regulation of sensations, will be discussed.

Chapter 5

# The role of music and rhythm in the development, integration and repair of the self

Eimir McGrath

Music and rhythm are an intrinsic part of being human, and we are surrounded by the rhythms of life that create an intrapersonal and interpersonal harmony essential for healthy growth and development. Each individual's capacity for social interaction is shaped by the earliest experiences of synchrony with the primary caregiver, where healthy attachment is formed through physiological and emotional regulation, the harmonic state of homeostasis. The biological functioning that is responsible for achieving and maintaining homeostasis is mainly controlled by the more primitive parts of the brain, the brainstem and cerebellum. Where adverse life events negatively impact on the ability to regulate both physiologically and emotionally, therapeutic interventions that are grounded in music and rhythm can support and enhance the growth, integration and repair of the self.

Music is a fundamental means of expression and communication that does not rely on verbal language or written signs. It is estimated that man first began to make music approximately 50,000 years ago, when communities were formed and began to 'symbolize, paint, speak and form kinship systems that held communities together' (Brandt, 2009: 31). Lee and Schögler (2009) define music as sound created by human action, engaging physiological, muscular, neural and behavioural systems in a creative act of expression. The most fundamental musical instrument is the human voice, and singing arose from the articulation of the voice into stable tones and intervals, linking the emotions of the breath with the rhythm of the body's movement (ibid.). Music is all-encompassing in its engagement of the whole person, the embodied self.

Rhythm surrounds us and can be understood as 'a strong regular repeated pattern of movement or sound' (*Oxford English Dictionary*). Environmentally, we experience the rhythm of day and night, the seasons, the ebb and flow of the tides. Intrapersonally, our world is full of rhythms, the breath, the heartbeat, the peristaltic action as food is digested. Interpersonally, we share the rhythms of interactions with others, a synchrony that evolves from the earliest experiences of interaction between the infant and the primary caregiver, experiences that begin *in utero*.

Both music and rhythm are innate mechanisms of each person's 'being in the world', contributing to the embodied presence of self that is central to existence.

However, embodied presence cannot be thought of in isolation. The human brain has evolved as a social entity: it is 'hard-wired' to interact with others, and recent advances in neuroscience have demonstrated how brain growth and development can only occur through a strong foundation in interpersonal relationships (Trevarthen, 1993; Cozolino, 2006; Schore, 2012; Siegel, 2012).

Rhythm and musicality are contained in the very first relationship, between the infant and the primary caregiver, providing the infant with a level of attunement and reciprocity that allows for healthy growth and development. Through the primary caregiver attuning to and regulating the infant's emotional states within the relationship, the infant gradually learns how to regulate his or her emotional states (Schore, 1994). These early rhythms of attuned relationship are the focus of this chapter, along with reference to the more primitive brain structures that are responsible for maintaining homeostasis, that state of being that provides internal stability and harmony and allows for healthy interaction with the outside world. The value of music and rhythm is explored as means of regaining homeostasis where the ability to regulate emotions has faltered, or as means of providing a reparative experience where the potential for emotional regulation has never been fully integrated by the self. Rhythmic communications at the start of life are intimately connected to the neurobiological structures that ensure physiological and emotional well-being (Cozolino, 2006; Trevarthen, 2009). By examining these elements, it is possible to have a deeper understanding of how the therapist can facilitate healing and growth through the rhythms and musicality of the therapeutic relationship. By the therapist using his or her own attuned presence, and also through the use of music and rhythm in activities, there is the potential to awaken the fundamental sense of connection vital for homeostasis and growth that is innate in each one of us.

Several strands have been identified that will now be examined in greater depth. First, the process of attachment will be discussed as the underpinning of all human growth and development. Second, the neurobiological aspects of emotional regulation, primarily based in the most primitive part of the brain, will be discussed. Third, through the use of a clinical case example, these elements will be brought from abstract theoretical discussion to live engagement, with suggestions for applying theory to practice throughout the developmental lifespan.

## The rhythm and musicality of attachment

Neuroscientist Colwyn Trevarthen emphasizes the importance of the musicality of early interactions in the attainment and maintenance of homeostasis. He states, 'infants are actually born with playful intentions and sensitivity to the rhythms and expressive modulations of a mother's talk and her visible expressions and touches' (2009: 58). His research over the past two decades confirms the vital importance of the rhythmic and melodic properties contained within the communication of dynamic mental states, and the building of shared narratives of experience. These are integral parts of the building blocks of relationship, and consequently of neural growth. In conjunction with researcher Niki Powers, Trevarthen's study of the emotions contained in early human vocal engagement determined that, 'a baby starts the journey an *innately musical/poetical being*, moving and hearing with pulse and rhythm, immediately sensitive to the harmonies and discords of human expression, in the Self and in companionship with close Others' (2009: 209; italics in original).

The musicality and rhythm contained within the early interactions and vocal conversations (protoconversations) between infant and caregiver are fundamental components in the development of attunement and, consequently, regulation and homeostasis (Trevarthen, 1979, 2009; Schore, 1994). When these are attained, there is the optimal opportunity for healthy growth and development to follow. Without adequate regulation allowing homeostasis to be achieved, growth and development are likely to be compromised.

As musicality and rhythm are such an intrinsic part of the creation of a 'we-ness' between two people, that early experience of primary intersubjectivity (Trevarthen, 2006), it follows that they offer a powerful means of intervention psychotherapeutically. Relationship-building between therapist and client can be assisted in a very fundamental way. For a client who has experienced a life event that has interfered with his or her ability to emotionally self-regulate, the use of rhythm and music can offer a means of providing external regulation until the client's own inner resources have been repaired. For clients who have experienced relational trauma and have perhaps never known a secure attachment, rhythm and music can be used to replicate, in a developmentally appropriate way, those building blocks of relationship that may have been missed in infancy and early childhood.

This very close link between internal biological rhythms and the attuned rhythms of intersubjectivity needs to be understood for full appreciation of the power of music and rhythm when used in a therapeutic setting. The biological rhythms that are shared between an infant and mother have their roots in the prenatal environment of the womb. The intrauterine environment of auditory, vibratory, proprioceptive and kinaesthetic stimuli provides the earliest form of attunement (Trevarthen, 1993). At a prenatal level, a synchronicity is already being created between mother and foetus through the shared experience of these biological and physical rhythms. The mother's heartbeat, breathing, the bodily actions of everyday life such as walking and the act of speech, all provide an interweaving of rhythm and movement that shapes early experience.

Mothers' brains are designed to be activated by the sights, sounds and smells of their newborn infants, creating the state of maternal preoccupation necessary for attunement to develop. Maestripieri (1999) states that evolution may have designed this shift as a purposeful maternal regression to more primitive modes of communication, allowing for a better connection with her newborn. Even these earliest of human interactions start to shape the social brain, and, as the primitive mechanisms that are responsible for ensuring survival all come into play, patterns of relating are being created at a neuronal level (Hughes, 2007). Thus, the experiences assimilated form the template upon which future interpersonal interactions will be based. As already discussed, the rhythm and musicality inherent in these very early communications play a vital role in physiological and emotional regulation and 'set the stage for the social regulation of biological processes throughout life' (Cozolino, 2006: 115). Consequently, coping and defence mechanisms will reflect these early patterns. It is at this primitive level that therapeutic intervention can either reinforce and reactivate healthy mechanisms where the client is under stress and needs external regulatory help, or can provide an experience of attunement and regulation to create new templates where previous ones were dysfunctional. Rhythm and music are fundamental pathways to achieving these aims.

Even before birth, the foetus is responding to the emotional states of the mother via the transmission of her neurochemicals through the placenta. For example, a chronically highly stressed mother will transmit increased cortisol levels to her unborn child, bringing about brain changes that increase the child's sensitivity to stimuli that startle or trigger a fear response (Bergman *et al.*, 2010). In situations of conflict where vocal patterns linked to aggression or fear are heard by the unborn baby, it is quite likely that neuronal connections are already being created within the baby's brain, causing a heightened reflexive response to this combination of increased cortisol level and voice patterns of similar pitch and intensity (ibid.). Consequently, at birth, the baby is already hypersensitive to experiencing a stress response in certain environmental situations. If the infant is repeatedly exposed to such experiences, a chronic state of hyperarousal is likely to develop, and a stressed mother becomes even more misattuned as her baby responds with alarm rather than pleasure to the mother's interactions. However, owing to the plasticity of the infant brain, new neuronal connections can be made as mother (or primary caregiver) and infant engage with each other face to face, in the rhythm of their shared communication that, as Winnicott (1953) says, is 'good enough'. This is a repair that can also be replicated in therapy (Cozolino, 2002).

Recent research regarding the use of music and rhythm in the hospital care of premature infants and neonates has indicated that there can be significant gains in infant well-being. Anecdotal evidence suggests that outcomes can be much more positive when music and meaningful noise are provided by a caregiver for infants in neonatal intensive care units. Research undertaken by Loewy *et al.* (2013) demonstrated changes in cardiac and respiratory function, feeding behaviours and sucking patterns, and increased periods of quiet alertness in preterm infants who were provided with a range of music and meaningful sound interventions. Shoemark *et al.* (2015) propose that the use of music as an integral part of neonatal intensive care can help promote sensory system maturation, reduce the impact of environmental stresses, facilitate transitioning between different physiological states, promote attachment and facilitate neurological development. Although this is a very new field of research, and further studies are needed to confirm these findings, there are enough indicators present to confirm the enormous benefit of using music for physiological and emotional calming of the newborn, as well as supporting healthy development. Perhaps the most powerful musical instrument for a newborn infant is the sound of the primary caregiver's voice. Trevarthen points out that, 'Infants certainly begin life with a well functioning awareness of the sounds of another person's feelings in the voice, especially for that uniquely known other person, the mother, whose voice has familiar and preferred qualities learned before birth' (2005: 69).

Malloch (1999) demonstrated that, in protoconversations, mothers and infants mutually adjust the pulse of their vocalizations and vary the quality of their expression systematically in order to produce a narrative lasting tens of seconds. During these protoconversations, they can respond synchronously or alternately and gradually develop a co-ordinated timing. Interactions become progressively more complex and lively, and, as the infant matures, the protoconversations become faster, with a wider range of rhythms and qualities of expression (Trevarthen, 1979, 1993, 2009a).

Through initially infantilizing their rhythm of speech, slowing down and engaging in a more melodic use of voice, narrative patterns are built by the primary caregiver, and the infant begins to predict and anticipate as these narrative patterns are repeated over and over again. This mode of communication, previously known as 'motherese', is now generally labelled as infant-directed speech. To the infant, the emotional content, his or her inner experience and the external reciprocal expression of emotion contained in each interaction become more and more predictable and understandable as healthy attachment is formed. Cozolino (2002) speaks of the power of face-to-face interactions, activating the infant's sympathetic nervous system and increasing oxygen consumption and energy metabolism, with the simultaneous production and availability of norepinephrine, endorphins and dopamine enhancing the child's energy and pleasure. The cascade of biochemical processes that arise from the physical and emotional interactions in the primary caregiver–infant dyad stimulate the growth of neural connections (Schore, 1997), enabling both physiological and emotional development. This neurobiological process will be explored in greater depth later.

Where attunement is inadequate, the subsequent effects on an infant are inevitably negative. Where basic rhythms of interaction have not been experienced, the infant's inner emotional world is adversely affected, and the expression of emotions is compromised, as is the ability to make meaning out of others' communications of emotion. Where an infant experiences ongoing episodes of relational misattunement by either an abusive caregiver or a preoccupied, dissociative caregiver, whose own experiences of trauma are unresolved, the normal development of the sense of self can be undermined, and, consequently, relational trauma can ensue. Not only are the infant's expressions of emotion not adequately and accurately mirrored in the shared narrative, but the misattuned communications initiated by the caregiver are confusing. Consequently, there is a drastic loss of the experience of effectiveness of the infant's emotional and communicative responses (Fonagy et al., 2004). Human infants have an exceptionally long period of dependence that requires intensive parenting, and, during these early years, there is enormous plasticity of the brain, as it quadruples in size between birth and 6 years. Consequently, the effects of emotional unavailability, misattunement, trauma and neglect can be enormous. If the rhythms of interaction and the musicality of early communications are missing or distorted, the long-term effect can be devastating, both relationally, in terms of self-regulation, and in the overall growth and development of the brain.

A closer look at the neurobiological processes that underpin the development of healthy attachment through affect regulation will provide a deeper understanding of the effect of relational trauma on the developing brain, and how this can have long-standing repercussions in the child's life.

## The neurobiology of attachment, regulation and communicative musicality

In a neurosequential model of brain development, the brain is divided into four main areas that are all interconnected: the brainstem, the diencephalon, the limbic system and the neocortex. This is a 'bottom–up' model of the brain that recognizes the evolutionary development from the most primitive, least complex structure of the brainstem, through the increasing complexity of the diencephalon and then the limbic system, to the most evolved part of the brain, the neocortex. With each level, the structure, function and cellular organization increase in complexity. When brain development and function are being considered, it is important to point out that the binary division between brain and body is really only a phenomenon found in anatomy textbooks. The historic notion that the brain is the controller of the body has long been disproved in favour of an understanding of the nervous system as being an integrated, embodied system that provides for a multidirectional flow of information, action and reaction (Siegel, 2007). Similarly, to divide the brain into specific areas of function is overly simplistic, as the interconnectivity within the brain is infinitely more complex than the historic belief that it can be rigidly mapped into discrete sites for specific tasks.

With this in mind, the role of music and rhythm will be discussed in relation to the more primitive parts of the brain and autonomic nervous system, with the focus on the more somatosensory aspects of regulation (although both music and rhythm obviously impact on the whole nervous system in a much more complex web of interconnectivity at all levels). These are the parts of the brain that are primarily responsible for maintaining physiological homeostasis and are an intrinsic part of emotional regulation. For the purpose of this chapter, homeostasis can be defined as 'a harmoniously balanced autonomic nervous system [that] responds to a situation as a function of the intensity of affective expression that would be considered appropriately within normal limits' (Montgomery, 2013: 35). The autonomic nervous system has multiple interconnections with the limbic system and plays a fundamental role in providing defence mechanisms for the individual. When the autonomic nervous system works in harmony, homeostasis

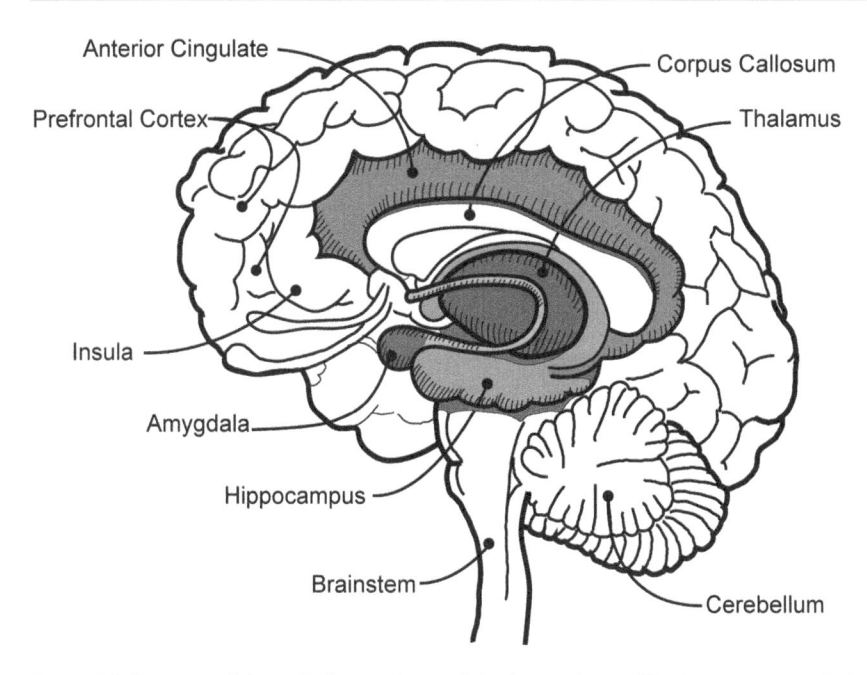

*Figure 5.1* Diagram of the right hemisphere of the human brain. The lower areas include the cerebellum and the brainstem; the central areas include the limbic regions (amygdala, hippocampus) and thalamus; the upper areas include the cortical regions. The insula is beneath this medial surface
Source: Siegel, 2012. © 2012 Mind Your Brain, Inc. Used with permission. All rights reserved

is achieved and maintained. This is what neuroscientist and psychiatrist Daniel Siegel (2012: 281) refers to as 'the "window of tolerance", in which various intensities of emotional arousal can be processed without disrupting the functioning of the system'.

## The brainstem

The brainstem is formed of the pons, the medulla and the midbrain (tectum and tegmentum). It connects the spinal cord with the cerebrum, and its main functions are networking between the cerebral cortex, the thalamus and the cerebellum; relaying sensation from the body to the thalamus; and sending messages from the cortex to the body. The brainstem provides the vital life-supporting autonomic functions of the peripheral nervous system. The pons contains nuclei that deal primarily with eye movement, facial expression and sensation, posture and equilibrium, hearing, taste, swallowing, bladder control, sleep and respiration. The medulla is responsible for the control of autonomic nervous activity, regulating respiration, heart rate, blood pressure and digestive processes. Within the midbrain, the tectum controls auditory and visual responses, and the tegmentum controls motor functions and regulates awareness and attention, as well as some autonomic functions. The emotion-mediating neurochemical systems all converge in the periaqueductal gray (PAG), the gray matter contained in the tegmentum. This core is sensitive to the positive affect communicated by others and triggers the release of reward-giving neurochemicals, as well as co-ordinating patterns of cardiovascular, respiratory, motor and pain modulatory responses to stimuli. It is also involved in defence mechanisms of the flight/freeze response to fear (Trevarthen, 2009; Benarroch, 2012).

## The cerebellum

The cerebellum is involved in the maintenance of balance and posture, co-ordination of voluntary movements, and motor learning (adapting and fine tuning to make movements more accurate). It is an intrinsic part of the system that leads from the perception of an action to the motor planning of that same action. It appears to provide the basic mirroring that is then linked to the emotional and cognitive processing inherent in the action (the somatosensory cortex is responsible for integration of the sensory, visceral and motor aspects of experience). Panksepp and Trevarthen (2009: 115) discuss the development of social communication through resonation with the intentions and feelings of others, 'probably by intrinsic affective systems situated much lower than the neocortex'. They describe this emotional awareness of both self and the other as the motivator of sociocultural existence and of 'each individual's urge from infancy to learn cultural skills, including those of language' (ibid.).

The sensory and motor capacities that create the human ability to communicate, along with the ability to emotionally regulate, are all situated subcortically. Even the earliest of human interactions start to shape the social brain, and, as the primitive mechanisms that are responsible for ensuring survival all come into play, patterns of relating are being created at a neuronal level (Cozolino, 2006; Hughes, 2007; Panksepp and Trevarthen, 2009).

These combined processes that involve the most primitive parts of the brain for emotional and physiological regulation, the building of relationships through early attachment experiences and the experiences of safety or otherwise, all combine to make us who we are. Porges states that, 'These psychological–physiological interactions are dependent on the dynamic bidirectional communication between peripheral organs and the central nervous system connecting the brain with these organs' (2009a: 28). He speaks of the neural circuits that mediate between body states and brainstem structures, not only promoting feelings but also enabling mental and psychological processes to influence body states and 'to color, and, at times, to distort our perceptions of the world' (ibid.). Through the development of his polyvagal theory (2007), a model of neural regulation of the autonomic nervous system, he has created a means of understanding the complexity of this system that is primarily one of safety seeking. It is beyond the scope of this chapter to explore Porges's theory in any detail, but a basic understanding will be outlined as it pertains to safety seeking, social connection and achieving physiological and emotional regulation.

The polyvagal system can be considered to have two main divisions, the defensive system and the social engagement system. The defensive system can be further divided into two subsystems, the domain of mobilization, including the fight/flight response that is controlled by the sympathetic nervous system, and the domain of immobilization, which triggers decreased muscle tension, decreased metabolic activity and possibly fainting and is controlled by the parasympathetic nervous system (2009: 39). This is the dorsal vagal system and it is unmyelinated – the most primitive part of the system. It is important to note that the type of freezing behaviour that requires increased muscle tension to inhibit movement comes under the first category of mobilization (the child is outwardly focused). So, a child in a state of frozen watchfulness is actually in mobilization mode; if that child then goes into a dissociative state in order to survive (the child is now inwardly focused), the immobilization domain has been activated (Porges, 2009b).

The myelinated ventral vagus, which is the most evolved, is the core of the social engagement system where facial expressions, human voice and head gesture are connected with the heart and heart rate variability, and all contribute towards an empathic awareness of others. This subsystem fosters calm behavioural states and dampens the hypothalamic pituitary adrenal (HPA) axis, which controls stress responses. This is the inhibition of the fight/flight mechanism of the sympathetic nervous system and is known as the vagal brake. It enables the individual to engage or disengage and to promote self-soothing behaviours and calm states. This system begins to develop at around 24 weeks' gestation, and development continues during the first year of life, with the myelination of the ventral vagus complex occuring rapidly in the last trimester of pregnancy and in the first few months after birth. If the infant's environment is one of constant threat and stress, the dorsal vagus complex is triggered to a degree that interferes with the myelination of the ventral vagus complex. Consequently, if homeostasis is challenged because of continually stressful environmental factors and inadequate, misattuned caregiving, the infant will be unable to successfully activate the vagal brake, which will compromise his ability to engage in social interactions. This can have an ongoing detrimental effect, not only on the growing child's ability to socialize, but also on the development of the child's brain architecture (Porges, 2007).

Porges introduced the notion of neuroception (2003), the non-conscious risk assessment that constantly evaluates what is safe, dangerous or life threatening, triggering or inhibiting defence strategies, to explain this process of seeking homeostasis in the underlying drive for survival.

By linking all of these elements of early attachment and interaction, safety and threat evaluation, along with the social engagement system, it is easy to understand how early experiences can create an expectation of the world's safety or otherwise. How those experiences are managed can profoundly influence our way of 'being in the world'. As has been demonstrated, the rhythm and musicality of the world in which we live and interact play a fundamental part in the achieving and maintaining of a level of homeostasis that allows healthy growth and development. Rhythm and music are vital tools in providing a therapeutic environment that can facilitate this process.

## Creating the dance of music and rhythm in therapy

At the start of all therapeutic engagements, one of the primary objectives is to ensure that soothing can take place, whether the client has the capacity to self-soothe or needs the therapist to be the 'external regulator'. By awakening the innate, primitive drive to respond to music and rhythm as regulatory mechanisms, soothing can be achieved regardless of the age or developmental stage of the client. Finding the appropriate tools for exploring rhythm and music will ensure that this can happen.

At all developmental stages, the empathic attunement of the therapist is the principal tool, as interactions are modulated to produce rhythmic experiences of intersubjectivity, thus helping the person towards a state of homeostasis, Siegel's 'window of tolerance'. From this position, emotional exploration can happen, whether that is symbolically through play, through creating a narrative with words or through embodied action whether the client is a young child, or where the level of trauma is significantly interfering with the ability to relate in any other way. Schögler and Trevarthen have researched the connection between singing, dancing and attunement, stating:

> Of all the ways we human beings share company, and communicate being alive, active and aware in our intricately mobile bodies, singing and dancing, the breath and activity of music, are the most elemental and persuasive. [...] There are messages in the polyrhythmic way our two-legged bodies move with the pulse and accents that can be varied to express the subtleties of will and consciousness to others.
>
> (2007: 281)

In these polyrhythmic communications within therapeutic interventions, there are some commonalities that can be identified and incorporated, regardless of the developmental stage of the client:

- Simple rhythmicity can be built into any activity wherever possible, whether it is in the therapist's use of voice or in his or her bodily actions.
- Repetition is vital. The more an interaction based on attuned regulation is experienced through the primitive relational systems embedded in rhythm and musicality, the stronger the building of new, healthier neuronal connections.
- Mirroring should be inbuilt also, trying to create face-to-face interaction wherever possible and appropriate. This can be done, not only through these

interactions, but also through organized movement activities to enhance the natural embodied mirroring that occurs as therapist and client communicate.

Rhythm and music can be used to soothe from states of both hyperarousal and hypoarousal, either calming or enlivening, but in each case with the therapist being very mindful to meet clients where they are at in order to initiate and maintain the communication. This constancy of attunement is essential to ensure that, when organized activities are being used, they do not become mechanical, meaningless exercises. In practice, the use of music and rhythm is interwoven within the therapeutic process, as can be seen in the following vignettes. Three vignettes will be presented, providing clinical examples of the inclusion of rhythm and musicality in therapy sessions at three different developmental levels: early childhood, adolescence and adulthood. (Each vignette is a compilation of several cases, in order to protect the confidentiality of the work.)

### Early childhood: Peter

Peter, a 3-year-old boy who had experienced a chaotic and unpredictable infancy and several short-term foster placements in the second year of his life, was struggling hugely with emotional regulation, which led to frequent 'meltdowns' with his long-term foster carers. His ability to engage in a playful way was seriously compromised by the overactively engaged mobilization system, which led him to play too aggressively with other children. He was constantly in a state of hyperarousal, unable to relax or allow his attention to be held for long enough in order to interact meaningfully either with the people around him or with his environment. It could be presumed that his experience of misattunement had been deeply confusing, and he perceived threat to be inherent in any interaction. As a result, he was physiologically unable to activate his social engagement system. In this case, working together therapeutically with both Peter and his foster parents was an integral part of the therapy, as he needed to have a reparative experience of a primary caregiver who could meet his emotional needs on a continuous basis, not just in the therapeutic hour. Consequently, nurturing and regulating games introduced during therapy could be carefully amalgamated into his home life.

Following the creation of a ritualized start to every session – the same welcome song, the same very simple jumping game using mats as stepping stones and large beanbags as safe islands to dive into – a series of other activities that would replicate very early infant interactions were gradually introduced. Such focused, large motor activities at the beginning of sessions gave him the opportunity to release the fight/flight energy that was contained in his body

> in a manner that allowed the reward system in his brain to become engaged, as the emphasis was on safety and containment. This provided a 'breathing space' into which nurturance could be introduced. Simple interactions between himself and his foster mother began to be used, where she replicated the maternal preoccupation that newborns usually experience. Cradling games – rocking together to the tune of a lullaby or his foster mother's singing – gave her the opportunity to gaze into his eyes and use her voice in the musical protoconversational tone usually reserved for tiny babies. More active rocking games such as 'Row, row, row your boat' were included as he began to be able to regulate his physiological arousal levels enough to play without becoming hyperaroused. As attunement began to develop, physical mirroring games were played, where his foster mother used facial expressions and gestures for him to copy, moving from simply 'sharing a smile' to gradually introducing very basic movement games, for example, both pretending to be sleepy, grumpy, surprised etc., with his foster mother using rhythmic movement wherever possible, initiating a shared dance. Action songs that invited the mirroring of gestures were used. A repertoire of predictable emotional communications and expressions was being built, all within an attuned manner that allowed Peter's social engagement system to be activated. Neuronal patterns were being created that came from an experience of nurturance rather than confusion, and existing patterns based on the unpredictability of another's responses were being extinguished and replaced.

With young children, nursery rhymes and songs that require mirroring of either gross or fine motor actions are invaluable, as they provide an embodied form of attunement. Such movements contain the vital elements of simple rhythm and repetition that build a sense of predictability and, consequently, safety and security, provided they are introduced and used in an attuned way. With older children, adolescents and adults, rhythmic movement can be introduced through activities such as simple sequences of progressive muscle relaxation, moving together to music (this can be anything along the continuum from small, simple hand movements to moving around the room), safe/self-massage and rhythmic body tapping. Any use of safe physical contact between therapist and client must, of course, be very carefully considered as to whether it is appropriate or not, especially where there has been trauma and abuse.

Other activities that can encourage the development of attunement and regulation through rhythm include 'passing' games, throwing a ball or any other object, where the rhythm of turn-taking is made concrete. This is a universally applicable activity. It is just as comfortable to engage a 3-year-old as it is to engage an adolescent or

## Adolescence: Rosie

Fourteen-year-old Rosie was referred for therapy because of her ongoing generalized anxiety, which was negatively impacting on her ability to manage daily life. School attendance was problematic, as any social engagement with peers triggered a stress response very much embedded in the sympathetic nervous system, causing her to experience feelings of panic and the need to flee. She consequently had very little energy and was constantly fatigued. The underlying cause of her distress emerged as therapy progressed: she had experienced a period of severe verbal bullying 2 years previously that had never been fully processed or resolved in a way that validated her emotional pain and soothed her fear of victimization and rejection. Our very first interactions centred on the recognition of her heightened physical stress as she sat in the room, close to tears and wringing her hands, with every muscle in her body tensed for flight as she perched precariously on the edge of the sofa.

I offered a selection of theraputties, malleable lumps of a plastic compound with different degrees of resistance, usually used in physiotherapy. I invited Rosie to test these, finding the one that best matched her stressful need to wring and squeeze. She chose the one that provided most resistance, and we both acknowledged how much energy was expended in the expression of her distress as she rhythmically squeezed and stretched the theraputty. I mirrored her movements as I joined in the activity. As the session progressed, attention was drawn to the gentle rocking motion of Rosie's body that had unconsciously begun. I suggested we tense and release other muscle groups/body parts in time with the squeezing and stretching of the theraputty, allowing the rocking to take on a consciously soothing rhythm. Gradually, Rosie's body began to relax. This technique was built on over subsequent sessions, reducing muscle tension with rhythmic hand and body movement, slowly stylizing the movements to create a seated dance to one of her favourite melodies that she identified as having a calming effect. All this took place from the safety of the sofa, where cushions, soft toys and a fluffy blanket provided a nurturance space that she could sink into, reminiscent of her very secure early childhood. A psycho-educational approach was used concurrently, so that Rosie would also have a cognitive understanding of how her brain and body were reacting to stress and fear. This had the effect of both providing reassurance that her reactions were understandable and also providing justification to engage in an activity that might otherwise be difficult for a self-conscious teenager. A ritual was thus created that established a coping technique that could be used to re-awaken Rosie's ability to self-soothe and emotionally regulate whenever she began to experience stress. It provided the vital basis for safety, containment and emotional regulation, so that the exploration of Rosie's distress could take place, which eventually led to the reduction of her anxiety and the re-establishment of a healthy social engagement system.

adult, where the therapist can provide a physical, regulatory accompaniment to conversation. A similar regulatory effect can be attained by offering play-dough, clay or any malleable object for the client to manipulate as they engage with the therapist. The resulting hand movements, as the object is manipulated, invariably become attuned to the client's own internal rhythm, as with Rosie.

### Adulthood: Helen

Helen's childhood and adolescence had been shaped by the relational trauma she had experienced within the family setting, where her single father had struggled with addiction and mental health issues following the death of her mother when Helen was an infant. She had survived the lack of consistent, attuned parenting by withdrawing into her own world, dissociating whenever the physical and emotional environment became overwhelming. As a young adult, she found it extremely difficult to form healthy, lasting relationships because of her inner sense of emptiness and worthlessness. Over a period of several years, Helen was able to engage therapeutically in the process of emerging from a position of emotional non-integration, through the grieving process for the loss of the possibility of a loving, attuned parent, to the integration of a sense of self that she could accept as a loveable and loving young woman. On this journey, creative approaches were frequently used to explore those aspects of her early life experience that were essentially wordless and to create opportunities for empathic attunement that could be reparative. Swaying to music, mirroring each other's movements, provided an experience of physical attunement that had been absent for her. The rhythmic interaction therapeutically replicated the reflective presence of a curious, attentive caregiver who offers emotional warmth in the to and fro of communication.

Children's storybooks that used rhythmic, repetitive language were carefully chosen and read, not only for the value of the musicality contained but also for the therapeutic message embedded within the story. Themes such as being lost and found, having overwhelming worries that sought resolution, and trying to find a sense of self were dominant. Together, we created a library of books that the little Helen would have enjoyed. This served several purposes: it provided the array of therapeutic themes; it also provided the innate sense of rhythm and musicality upon which attuned communication is built; and, equally importantly, through the selection of books that reflected developmental growth, it recreated a historic sequence for Helen. The library provided a metaphoric journey from infancy through to late childhood, creating an opportunity to build a sense of self in a safe, contained manner.

Reading aloud stories that contain repetitive phrases and singing songs with repetitive words also provide regulatory, rhythmic input. With children, this is very much part of a normal play repertoire. The same effect can be gained with adolescents and adults through the creation or use of poetry, the introduction of appropriate music into the session, or even through the introduction of a 'nostalgia' session, exploring children's rhymes and songs that may have been positively experienced at an earlier stage, or perhaps choosing a collection that the client perceives as appealing to a young child.

The use of musical instruments, either to create music or accompany movement, is invaluable as a means of communication as well as expression. Using instruments in 'call-and-answer'-type games provides an opportunity for therapist and client to mirror each other's rhythms, as well as providing the therapist with a means of regulating the client's arousal state through the rhythms created. This is particularly useful for young children. Fast, loud music-making can be gradually slowed and calmed, and, conversely, a child can be led to a state of optimal arousal from hypoarousal through increasing vitality and intensity in the rhythms and melodies created. Tapping out rhythms of favourite songs may be a means of engaging an adolescent or adult in a similar activity, leading on to creating a personal rhythm that is pleasing to the client.

The rhythmic use of breathing can also act as a regulator for children and adults alike. The younger the client, the more this will have to be embodied in a very concrete way, for example through blowing bubbles, playing a wind instrument such as a recorder or harmonica, or perhaps blowing a paper windmill. With older children and adults, a more abstract approach can be taken with the introduction of mindful breathing and relaxation and development of an awareness of bodily movements associated with the rhythm of breath. It is worth noting that adolescents and adults who are highly traumatized are most likely unable to use mental visualization, and a very concrete approach, along with careful monitoring, would be required.

## Conclusion

It seems that rhythmical qualities of the earliest interpersonal experiences become part of a deeply rooted knowledge of how to relate to other human beings, and these prelinguistic ways of being are awakened by shared music and rhythm. This is an inbuilt mechanism that can be accessed whenever an individual needs to emotionally regulate, either through self-soothing or with the support of the therapist, who can become 'external regulator'. Where someone has experienced life events that have had an adverse effect on their ability to cope, engaging in therapy provides support in attaining emotional regulation until resilience has been regained.

Thanks to the brain's plasticity, therapeutic engagement can also provide a reparative experience of attunement where there has been a history of relational trauma. In order for this to successfully come about, it is necessary for the therapist to have an understanding of the relational needs of the client, where early attachment has not provided a good enough grounding, and also a knowledge of the mechanisms that affect the ability to emotionally regulate. By taking a developmentally informed approach to the therapeutic relationship, not only can the missing elements of relationship be recognized, but developmentally appropriate interventions can be formulated. Music and rhythm are the fundamental constituents of an intersubjectivity upon which all relationship, and consequently therapy, is based. By a conscious inclusion of these constituents in the therapeutic process, emotional and physiological homeostasis can be attained, facilitating the development, integration and repair of the self.

## Key points

- Music and rhythm are intrinsically contained in all human interactions and are embedded in the developing brain prenatally.
- Both physiological and emotional regulation (homeostasis) depends upon the creation and maintenance of the rhythms and musicality of interpersonal relationships.
- The functions of the brainstem and cerebellum are largely responsible for the more primitive mechanisms that help achieve and maintain homeostasis.
- Through the attuned use of music and rhythm in the therapeutic process, emotional regulation can be supported where normal resilience has been affected by adverse life events.
- Reparative experiences of empathic attunement through the use of music and rhythm can bring about change at a neuronal level where there has been relational trauma.

## References

Benarroch, E. (2012). Periaqueductal gray. An interface for behavioural control. *Neurology*, *78*(3), 210–17.
Bergman, K., Sarkar, P., Glover, V., and O'Connor, T.G. (2010). Maternal prenatal cortisol and infant cognitive development: Moderation by infant–mother attachment. *Biological Psychiatry*, *67*(11), 1026–32.
Brandt, P.A. (2009). Music and how we became human – A view from cognitive semiotics. In S. Malloch and C. Trevarthen (eds) *Communicative Musicality. Exploring the basis of human companionship*. Oxford, UK: Oxford University Press.
Cozolino, L. (2002). *The Neuroscience of Psychotherapy*. New York: Norton.
Cozolino, L. (2006). *The Neuroscience of Human Relationships*. New York: Norton.
Fonagy, P., Gergely, G., Jurist, E., and Target, M. (2004). *Affect Regulation, Mentalization, and the Development of the Self*. London: Karnac.
Hughes, D. (2007). *Attachment Focused Family Therapy*. New York: Norton.
Lee, D., and Schögler, B. (2009). Tau in musical expression. In S. Malloch and C. Trevarthen (eds) *Communicative Musicality. Exploring the basis of human companionship*. Oxford, UK: Oxford University Press.

Loewy, J., Stewart, K., Dassler, A.M., Telsey, A., and Homel, P. (2013). The effects of music therapy on vital signs, feeding, and sleep in premature infants. *Pediatrics*, *131*(5), 902–18.
Malloch, S. (1999). Mother and infants and communicative musicality. *Musicae Scientae* (Special Issue 1999–2000), 29–57.
Maestripieri, D. (1999). The biology of human parenting: Insights from nonhuman primates. *Neuroscience & Behavioural Reviews*, *23*, 411–22.
Montgomery, A. (2013). *Neurobiology Essentials for Clinicians*. New York: Norton.
Panksepp, J., and Trevarthen, C. (2009). The neuroscience of emotion in music. In S. Malloch and C. Trevarthen (eds) *Communicative Musicality: Exploring the basis of human companionship*. Oxford, UK: Oxford University Press.
Porges, S. (2003). Social engagement and attachment. A phylogenetic perspective. *Annals of the New York Academy of Sciences*, *1008*, 31–47. Available at: www.psy.miami.edu/faculty/dmessinger/c_c/rsrcs/rdgs/attach/Porges_socialEngagement Attachment.pdf (accessed 30 August 2015).
Porges, S. (2007). The polyvagal perspective. *Biological Psychology*, *74*(2), 116–43. Available at: www.ncbi.nlm.nih.gov/pmc/articles/PMC1868418/ (accessed 4 September 2015).
Porges, S. (2009a). Reciprocal influences between body and brain development. In D. Fosha, D. Siegel and M. Solomon (eds) *The Healing Power of Emotion* (pp. 27–54). New York: Norton.
Porges, S. (2009b). The polyvagal theory: New insights into adaptive reactions of the autonomic nervous system. *Cleveland Clinical Journal of Medicine*, *76* (suppl. 2), S86–S90. Available at: www.ncbi.nlm.nih.gov/pmc/articles/PMC3108032/ (accessed 10 September 2015).
Powers, N., and Trevarthen, C. (2009). Voices of shared emotion and meaning: Young infants and their mothers in Scotland and Japan. In S. Malloch and C. Trevarthen (eds) *Communicative Musicality: Exploring the basis of human companionship* (pp. 209–40). Oxford, UK: Oxford University Press.
Schögler, B., and Trevarthen, C. (2007). To sing and dance together: From infants to jazz. In S. Bråten (ed.) *On Being Moved: From mirror neurons to empathy*. Amsterdam: John Benjamins.
Schore, A. (1994) *Affect Regulation and the Origin of the Self*. Mahwah, NJ: Erlbaum.
Schore, A. (1997). Interdisciplinary developmental research as a source of clinical model. In M. Moskowitz, C. Monk, C. Kaye and S. Ellman (eds) *The Neurobiological and Developmental Basis for Psychotherapeutic Intervention* (pp. 1–71). Lanham, MD: Jason Aronson.
Schore, A. (2012). *The Science of the Art of Psychotherapy*. New York: Norton.
Shoemark, H., Hanson-Abromeit, D., and Stewart, L. (2015). Constructing optimal experience for the hospitalized newborn through neuro-based music therapy. *Frontiers in Human Neuroscience*, *9*, article 487. Available at: http://journal.frontiersin.org/article/10.3389/fnhum.2015.00487/full (accessed 18 October, 2015).
Siegel, D. (2007). *The Mindful Brain*. New York: Norton.
Siegel, D. (2012). *The Developing Mind: How relationships and the brain interact to shape who we are* (2nd edn). New York: Guilford Press.
Trevarthen, C. (1979). Communication and co-operation in early infancy. A description of primary intersubjectivity. In M. Bulowa (ed.) *Before Speech: The beginning of human communication*. Cambridge, UK: Cambridge University Press.

Trevarthen, C. (1993). The self born in intersubjectivity: The psychology of an infant communicating. In U. Neisser (ed.) *The Perceived Self: Ecological and interpersonal sources of self knowledge*. Cambridge, UK: Cambridge University Press.

Trevarthen, C. (2005). Stepping away from the mirror: Adventures in companionship. Reflections on the nature and emotional needs of infant intersubjectivity. In C.S. Carter, L. Ahnert, K.E. Grossman, S.B. Hrdy, M.E. Lamb, S.W. Porges and N. Sachser (eds) *Attachment and Bonding: A new synthesis* (pp. 55–84). Dahlem Workshop Report 92. Cambridge, MA: MIT Press.

Trevarthen, C. (2006). The concepts and foundations of intersubjectivity. In S. Bråten (ed.) *Intersubjective Communication and Emotion in Early Ontogeny* (pp. 15–46). Cambridge, UK: Cambridge University Press.

Trevarthen, C. (2009). The functions of emotion in infancy. The regulation and communication of rhythm, sympathy, and meaning in human development. In D. Fosha, D. Siegel and M. Solomon (eds) *The Healing Power of Emotion* (pp. 55–85). New York: Norton.

Winnicott, D. (1953). Transitional objects and transitional phenomena: A study of the first not-me possession. *International Journal of Psychoanalysis*, *34*(2), 89–97.

# Chapter 6

# Being, becoming and healing through movement and touch

*Maggie Fearn and Pablo Troccoli*

This chapter introduces the fascinating story of how, *in utero* and during the first months after birth when our first sensory perceptions occur, we experience ourselves in the world through movement and touch. We explore how our earliest experiences model and shape the way we engage in relationship and environmental interactions, from early attachment and throughout our lives.

Through case study examples, we consider the impact of early developmental trauma and neglect on well-being across the lifespan. We examine how play therapy can support recovery by calming and reorganizing traumatized nervous system responses through movement and touch experiences. Particular attention is paid to the therapist's role and presence, the relational field and the therapeutic environment.

## Early development

> The nature and timing of our developmental experiences shape us.
> (Perry and Szalavitz, 2006: 98)

Layer upon layer of embodied experiences have formed our physiological constitution. Rather than being a linear process, our development spirals through time, each stage dependent on the previous and overlapping with the next in a wave-like motion (Stern, 1985; Bainbridge Cohen, 2012). Through sensing, feeling and action, we constantly and unconsciously express our very earliest experiences through our particular way of being in the world (Grof and Bennett, 1992; Levine and Kline, 2007; Bainbridge Cohen, 2012). It is not possible to consciously access and express preverbal autobiographical experience, because the language of preverbal memory comprises movement and sensory information clusters, situated in the nonverbal, right hemisphere of the brain. Schore (2005) tells us that the early-maturing right brain undergoes a growth spurt in the first 2 years, before the verbal left brain, and remains dominant for the first 3 years. The right hemisphere is predominant in processing sensory information and the development of the emotional and embodied self: 'The social experience-dependent maturation of the right brain in human infancy is equated with the early development of self' (Schore, 2005: 205). Thus, human infants primarily experience the world and communicate through sensory experience. We argue that movement and touch underpin the development of all the other senses, and the relevance of this for play therapy practitioners is explored in this chapter.

## Why movement? Why touch?

From our earliest single-cell beginnings, movement and touch are inseparable. Unicellular organisms are capable of sensing the direction of the gravity field, generating locomotion to adjust their body orientation in space and reaching out with their membrane receptors for vital environmental clues. The survival of the organism relies on the motility and sensitivity to touch of its receptors. Multicellular organisms are infinitely more complex, but their biological design is founded upon the same basic priorities (Vinnikov, 1974). From this perspective, at the time when human senses of taste, smell, hearing and vision are at early stages of development, movement and touch already inform sensory reception of stimuli, facilitating the recording of patterns and synaptic connection. Therefore, although movement is 'our first perception' (Bainbridge Cohen, 2012: 115), touch is embedded in it. Furthermore, if, as Bainbridge Cohen (2012) states, movement is also our first experience of learning, then early human development depends upon our 'tactile-kinesthetic bodies' (Sheets-Johnstone, 1998: 275).

In the first trimester, the fetus micro-moves in a sequence of pre-spinal movement patterns with different qualities, evocatively described as vibration, cellular breathing, sponging, pulsation and navel radiation (Brook, 2001; Bainbridge Cohen, 2012). Simultaneously, a set of primitive reflexes is developing within the neurological structures of the low and midbrain (Brook, 2001). These primitive reflexes provide the neurological impetus for more complex developmental movement patterns, which manifest during birth and infancy and which, in their turn, will be constantly informed and repatterned by successive environmental experiences through the lifespan.

## Movement, touch and emotional development

Survival of the infant depends on *in utero* development of the autonomic nervous system, which controls most of the involuntary visceral activities of the body (Schoenwolf *et al.*, 2009). 'At birth, for example, the brainstem areas responsible for regulating cardiovascular and respiratory function must be intact for the infant to survive, and any malfunction is immediately observable' (Perry, 2008: 97). The autonomic nervous system coordinates the processes necessary for our first vocal expression and movements involved in feeding, such as: oral reach, grasping, releasing, sucking and swallowing. Furthermore, its vast neurological networks will also orchestrate coordination of the chemical and mechanical transformations necessary for digestion, assimilation and elimination of wastes from our first nourishment.

Structurally, the autonomic nervous system includes the parasympathetic and sympathetic divisions and the exclusive neuronal enervation of the gastrointestinal tract. The neurological network of the gut is called the enteric nervous system. The vagus pair of cranial nerves are a fundamental part of the enteric nervous system. They exit the skull and meander around the body to enervate facial muscles, palate, throat, heart and lungs, liver, kidneys, pancreas and the entire gastrointestinal tract. Through the vagus nerves, the brainstem is informed about the infant's visceral state and, after exchanging this information with other feedback systems of the brain, delivers a modulating response. In infancy, visceral state activation, such as tiredness, hunger, thirst, being too hot or too cold, and need for defecation, is a demand that cannot be ignored or delayed without causing distress, which results in highly reactive, physiological arousal. The infant relies completely on the caregiver for recognition and actions to meet their needs and establish and maintain homeostasis, only gradually integrating the ability to self-regulate. Therefore, constantly monitoring, tracking and communicating sensory information, the autonomic nervous system weaves and wires the neurological infrastructure for relational and emotional development in the infant.

In this respect, the 'polyvagal theory' appears particularly relevant for understanding situations where early trauma, neglect or stress has disturbed the maturation of self-regulation processes that underpin normal development of socially adaptive and defensive behaviours (Porges 2003). Porges proposes that, in more advanced developmental stages, social engagement behaviours appear to continue to be driven by the body's visceral state. Humans need to maintain homeostasis in order to feel safe and to function well in relationship with others. If we do not feel safe, we become hypervigilant, shutting down the social engagement system and activating physiological arousal. This manifests in altered heart rate and breathing, shutdown of the digestive system and the activation of the defensive sympathetic fight or flight response, or the defensive parasympathetic shutdown or freeze response.

Porges suggests that, to calm the stress response, we can recruit the neural circuits that promote social behaviour through a variety of techniques that focus on safety: reducing the amount of stimulation in the environment, using calm intonation, listening, familiar faces, familiar people and careful touch (Dykema, 2006).

The skin is a specialized sensory organ, forming the external boundary of the human embryo, initially, *in utero*, a single cell layer thick (Schoenwolf *et al.*, 2009). The development of this semipermeable tissue into the main organ of the sense of touch progresses hand in hand with the maturation of the nervous system. Both the external layer of the skin (epidermis) and the brain, spinal cord and accessory nerves are derived from the same ectoderm cellular layer. The central nervous system develops as the gatherer, recorder and monitor of sensory information, and networking coordinator of motor responses, whereas the skin is situated at the periphery, mediating internal and external environmental relationship. In the light of their close embryological origin and their later reciprocal function, it might be useful to consider skin as a visible part of the nervous system, and to consider the central nervous system as the hidden side of the skin (Montagu, 1978).

Therefore, to touch someone is to be touched in return (Montagu, ibid.) and is an exquisitely sensitive act. The information exchanged in the act of touch is put in relationship with everything held within both nervous systems – we receive and respond to touch with our whole being, past and present. This reveals the potential therapeutic relevance of safe touch. Porges (2011) describes the need for a preamble to touch that prepares the nervous system for the encounter. Typically, in early attachment relationship, an attuned mother will use voice, gesture and face-to-face communication before touching the infant. 'Maternal sensitivity, therefore, acts as an external organizer of the infant's biobehavioral regulation' (Schore, 2005: 207).

The development of the organic foundations of an emotional life take place while the unborn child is receiving and sharing what the mother breathes, eats, drinks, thinks, voices and feels (Gerhardt, 2005; Sunderland, 2006; Brown, 2009). Neurologically, emotional development is synchronous with sensory discrimination. Panksepp and Biven (2012) describe how incoming motor-sensory information travels up the spinal cord and enters the periaqueductal grey region of the brainstem. From here, this information is differentiated into seven core affect systems that organize and hold the infant's potential for experiencing emotion. These potentialities manifest as curiosity; care and nurture; joy and play; fear; rage; panic at abandonment; and, in puberty, sexual curiosity and excitement. This affective potential is realized, for better or worse, via the attachment bond with the primary caregiver.

## Movement, touch and hearing

The first cranial nerves to show signs of maturation are the vestibulocochlear nerves, which will enervate the vestibular system and the hearing sense (Sampaio and Truwitt, 2001). In contrast with the optic nerves and sense of vision that will reach maturity by the third post-natal month, movement detection, the sense of hearing and related structures of the brainstem are fully developed by the middle of the ninth fetal month (Sampaio and Truwitt, 2001). The vestibular system, located in the inner ear, adds a new dimension to the spatial reality of the fetus. Now, not only can they move and their nervous system can continually develop in response to touch (feedback from their actions), but also, via the vestibular organs of balance, they can sense movements initiated by their environment and respond accordingly (Bainbridge Cohen, 2012).

Thus, *in utero*, in symbiotic relationship, the developing child has the capacity to resonate with, and move in relation to, the sound, vibrations and pulsations of their mother's heart rate, breathing pattern, emotions, voice and visceral movements, as well as the ability to detect changes in the mother's body position in space. The first environment of relationship is the living body of the mother: within this living environment, the nervous system of the baby develops and is imprinted with the primal neurological information that initially prefigures her unique way of perceiving and interacting with inner and outer worlds. *In utero* experiences establish patterns of interaction that develop, via the birth experience, into the post-natal attachment relationship.

## Movement, touch and post-natal attachment

Implicit memories are preconscious embodied experiences, embedded in the nervous system through repetition and association of moving, sensing, feeling and responding. The neurological systems that support implicit memory are thought to be functional from the last third of pregnancy (Schore, 2002; Siegel, 2012). Therefore, as newborns, we already carry within us an imprint of our *in utero* experiences (Grof and Bennett, 1992) and our birth experiences (Rank, 1993; McCarty, 2014).

As the fetus's development depends on the qualities of the *in utero* environment, so the newborn's survival depends on the care and synchronous attention of the mother (Schore, 2002). They need to re-establish connection with each other after birth through the mother's familiar movement qualities, emotional range and prosody – the music, tones and rhythms of her voice – and her unique style of touch (Schore, 2005; Porges, 2011). This very particular weave of movement, sound and touch forms the fabric of the child's first felt experience in the world and provides the context for development of co-regulation in the attachment relationship between the mother and child.

A child's healthy development is rooted in the belief that the world is a trustworthy place, that it is safe to feel, respond and to express big feelings, and that the caregiver will respond soon enough in a way that soothes, reassures and differentiates (Gerhardt, 2005; Porges, 2003). If the baby feels safe in a synchronous relationship where her basic needs are met, she will yield to the offered support, seek out sensory information and develop through an increasing repertoire of movement and sensory explorations in her environment (Bainbridge Cohen, 2012; Brook, 2001; Frank and La Barre, 2011).

Thus, our regulatory capacity is implicit, preconscious and preverbal. It is patterned in the somatosensory cortex and the early affective brain systems that inform the emotional and relational aspects of the limbic system. It follows that, provided we have integrated, healthy regulatory capacity, we can form and maintain human and environmental relationships that help us establish a consistent sense of self and make sense of and build on life's experiences.

## The impact of adverse experiences

Perry (2008: 93) defines trauma as 'an experience or pattern of experiences which activate the stress-response systems in such an extreme or prolonged fashion as to cause alterations in the regulation and functioning of these systems'. He defines neglect as 'the absence of an experience or pattern of experiences required to express an underlying genetic potential in a key developing neural system' (cited in Prasad, 2011: 2). He argues that the brain develops sequentially and is organized in hierarchical sequence, and that neurons and neural systems are use-dependent, that is, their development is driven by experience.

Therefore, developmental trauma or neglect is hardwired into the neural system at the time it occurs and becomes more embedded every time it reoccurs. The child will have an altered baseline homeostasis and will rarely experience an internal state of calm and rest. Even when removed from chaotic, violent or neglectful circumstances, the traumatized or neglected child may continue to perceive constant threat from the environment and will be unable to modulate the intense arousal of the stress response. Overreactive and hypersensitive, they may be extremely tense, with an increased startle response, disturbed emotional regulation, generalized or specific anxiety and abnormal cardiovascular regulation (Perry, 2004).

The stress-response state can manifest on a hyperaroused through to dissociative continuum, and different children have different adaptive styles to threat. Much depends on the characteristics of the original adverse circumstances, the degree of agency of the child and the degree of perceived threat: the hyperaroused child will respond from somewhere on the continuum of vigilance, resistance, defiance and aggression; on the other hand, the dissociative child will respond on the continuum of avoidance, compliance, dissociation and fainting (Perry, ibid.).

Neural systems can be repatterned precisely because they are designed to change in response to activity. Developmentally appropriate therapeutic interventions can make a difference, although some neural systems (brainstem and midbrain) are harder to influence than others (cortex). However, the impact of trauma and neglect on the lower brain regions can be mitigated through therapeutic relationship that addresses core regulation, replicating healthy early attachment experiences and giving the child, adolescent or adult repeated opportunities to experience internal rest and calm. Safety, predictability and nurturance are the key principles of core regulation (Rothschild, 2000; Perry, 2004), normally established *in utero* and in the earliest relational experiences of attachment during the first 2 years of life, when the brain is developing faster than at any other time.

Therefore, in cases of early developmental trauma or neglect, there is a need for carefully targeted therapeutic interventions that understand the nature and timing of the adversity the child has suffered, provide a secure and trustworthy relationship and a safe, predictable environment over a significant period of time, and use responsive, attuned movement, prosody and reassuring safe touch as primary modes of communication.

In play therapy, the child repatterns the nervous system by visiting a safe, undisturbed developmental stage previous to the trauma or neglect experiences, so that another way forward can be imagined and experienced in the safety of the metaphorical play environment and the therapeutic relationship. The metaphors and symbols of play – the 'as ifness' of it – coupled with the empathic, unconditional positive regard of an attuned therapeutic relationship provide safe distance that protects the child from overwhelm of traumatic re-experiencing (Prendiville, 2014a). Positive dyadic play is crucial to the development of the primary attachment relationship and can be replicated in the therapeutic relationship, providing a template for social engagement and interaction that can offer lifelong protection against isolation and the resulting panic, grief and fear (Panksepp and Biven, 2012). Furthermore, Perry (2008) insists that, although effective, one hour of therapy a week alone will not support lasting change. Children need to experience attuned, empathic and playful relationship little and often. He recommends involving key people in the child's life in a web of coordinated interactions and repeat experiences that cooperate to provide a consistent, caring and playful environment.

## Applications in play therapy

> Surely we need to look again at the question of emotional hunger?
> (Jennings, 2011: 126)

In her developmental play therapy model, Jennings (1999) takes a sequential approach to therapeutic interventions that can be corroborated by Perry's neurosequential model of therapeutics (Perry and Hambrick, 2006). Jennings (2011) describes the sensory, rhythmic and dramatic play that takes place between a mother and her unborn or newborn baby. Similarly to Brown (2009), Jennings (2011) proposes that a mother's play with her unborn child 'has a profound effect on the growth of the [baby's] brain' (Jennings, 2011: 33). An expectant mother's play, particularly rhythmic movement and touch experiences such as massage, finger drumming, playing of soothing music and rhythmic rocking, can decrease anxiety and stress hormone levels for the mother, simultaneously providing valuable soothing bodily experiences for the unborn and newborn child. In addition, Jennings (2011) proposes that an expectant mother's regular dialogue with her unborn and newborn child represents a dramatic playful interaction between them that facilitates early experiences of role-play, the beginning of reciprocity and the development of a caring, loving and predictable relationship that is at the core of healthy attachment.

These principles and techniques can be used successfully in play therapy with children, adolescents and adults to enhance and repair attachment, focusing on embodied experiences of sensory play and messiness, rhythmic play and ritual, and dramatic play and mimicry. Sensory play experiences involving touch and movement – such as gentle blowing; textures; smells; visual movement using colours; sucking and tasting; soothing sounds; listening and responding; loving gestures and prosody – all provide playful opportunities for human contact, a critical element in the attachment process (Harlow and Zimmerman, 1959; Booth and Jernberg, 2010; Jennings, 2011; Sori and Schnur, 2013; Whelan and Stewart, 2014).

Incorporating rhythmic play experiences, involving clapping, humming, chanting, drumming, singing, finger rhymes, rocking and rhythmic movement-based games, provides playful opportunities for both parents and therapists to provide positive safe touch and develop and strengthen a responsive relationship with the child, while simultaneously helping the child internalize and integrate a sense of repetition and predictability, qualities that have been identified as critical in the development of a secure attachment (Norton and Norton, 2008; Booth and Jernberg, 2010; Perry, 2000; Jennings, 2011).

Cattanach (1994), Gil (2010) and Jennings (2011) propose that facilitating dramatic play experiences for very young children, as well as for older clients who have suffered early developmental trauma, encourages the development of synchrony between parent and child, or therapist and client, another essential element in the attachment and healing process (Feldman, 2007). Jennings categorizes different play types: consonant play refers to playful experiences in which parent/therapist and child are engaged in the same activity. These range from simple movements such as dancing together or rocking while holding the child to gentle, affectionate, rough-and-tumble play. Echo play occurs when the child echoes the sounds and movements of the adult, and mimicry develops a reciprocal drama whereby the child imitates the adult and the adult imitates the child. Mirroring occurs when the child begins to imitate both actions and sounds and further develops when the child begins to initiate them.

Dramatic play enables the child to perform actions and observe their parent or therapist performing the same action, thus resulting in the activation of mirror neurons in the child's developing brain (Stamenov and Gallese, 2002; Rizzolatti *et al.*, 2006; Gallese, 2007). It is proposed that these mirror neurons contribute to a child's ability to understand the behaviours of others and 'thus play a role in how children learn about the world, how to act, and how to play' (Stagnitti, 2009: 62). This process is instrumental in the child's developing self-awareness, as illustrated in the following extract from a play therapist's notes:

> Session 7: Large inflatable ball . . . M (aged 7yrs) bounces it back and forth between us in different ways. Then belly rolling on the ball . . . I had to do it too. Then sitting on it and bouncing six times and rolling off . . . I had to do it too. This is somatic mirroring as it occurs in the early attachment relationship: she wants to see what she has just done. It is as if she is saying to me 'I don't know what I have done . . . You do it and I will see it. . . . I want to have a sense of what I feel from watching you.'
>
> Session 8: She bursts into the playroom and looks around. Speeding up, she picks up the cookery basket, sorts the things she wants and begins measuring, mixing and counting the ingredients, instructing me to do exactly what she did. Her hands are shaking slightly and she is very tense. I feel I have to get it right, that a lot depends on me being able to copy her exactly. I feel anxious, and I am aware I may be feeling her anxiety. Again I am her mirror, reflecting back to her, her inner state, and I am, in turn, able to calm her anxiety by

consciously slowing my own breathing, modulating my own feelings of anxiety and calming myself down.

(Fearn, 2015)

## The therapist's use of self

An integrative and humanistic play therapist approaches play therapy with deep curiosity about the child's experience of being in the world, as expressed through their play on a moment-by-moment basis. As well as the therapist drawing on the therapeutic powers of play (Schaefer and Drewes, 2014), considering the play environment and applying different theoretical approaches to therapeutic presence according to each child's needs, the therapist's curiosity is informed by study and observation of psychological and physiological development processes.

First-person experiential study of developmental movement patterns creates the possibility of an embodied understanding of another person moving. If I pay careful attention to my experience of myself in the world, I am aware of where I am, how I feel, what I do, how I do it and my effect on others: I am aware of my presence in relationship to the people I work with and care for. Exploring somatic principles of mirroring, movement of attention, sensing qualities of movement and careful observation of self and other helps to develop an ability to listen with the body and respond empathically. This supports effective nonverbal communication with the predominantly right-brain, infant state of being (Schore, 2011).

As well as somatic awareness, the therapist consistently uses techniques of non-intrusive responding, tracking and reflection throughout all the following case study sessions (Yasenik and Gardner, 2012).

## Using movement- and touch-based activities in psychotherapy across the lifespan

### Sally (aged 3 years)

Sally's mother, Tracey, said the pregnancy and birth were normal and she described an easy relationship with Sally within the context of a vibrant extended family. Sally's father came and went and was not involved in parenting. At 19 months old, when Sally's brother was born and hospitalized for several months, Sally was looked after at home by her grandparents and separated from her mother every day. She would cry a lot when Tracey left her and then calm down when she phoned. Her separation distress was activated, but the adults knew there was no danger, and she received a sensitive, reassuring response from her primary caregivers (Panksepp and Biven, 2012). Provided one of them was present, it seems that Sally was able to manage her fright and panic.

However, at 24 months, she was suddenly taken into hiding with her siblings, because her father attacked her mother in front of them. Tracey admitted enduring many months of this treatment, but she thought the children did not witness it up to this point in time, and she removed them to prevent it happening again. However, because of the co-regulatory process in the attachment relationship, Sally may have already been sensitized by, and internalized, the effect of her father's treatment of her mother, setting in motion a chronic stress response. Unfortunately, having to suddenly go into hiding activated Tracey's 'flight' system, and she was acutely anxious. It is likely that, at this point, Sally began to suffer mis-attunement, being out of sync with her mother and separated from the reassuring presence of her grandparents. The three key conditions for healthy play and development, which are safety, predictability and nurturance, were simultaneously denied to her. This would be traumatizing for such a young child, triggering dysregulation and exacerbating a chronic hyperaroused state of vigilance and resistance (Perry, 2004).

Intervention focused on three strands simultaneously:

1   establishing a rapport between the therapist and Sally's mother and inviting her into the play therapy sessions with Sally;
2   establishing a sense of safety and predictability and at first limiting the play materials in the playroom to avoid overstimulation;
3   working in a threesome with the mother and child together to re-establish their early attachment bond through playful communication.

It was necessary for the therapist to be focused on the mother–child relationship, to model non-intrusive responsiveness and accurate timing in following the child's play, and, seamlessly, to step in and pick up interaction with Sally when her mother lost concentration and dropped her connection with her.

Sally is extremely anxious at the start of the first three sessions. She clings on to Tracey and says 'Take me home'. Tracey talks to her and tries to reason with her, but this does not work. I encourage Tracey to soothe Sally by holding her close, rocking her and stroking her hair, murmuring to her. As Tracey slows down and focuses intently on Sally's well-being, using the rhythm of rocking and stroking, and the gentleness of her touch and her tone of voice, both Tracey and Sally relax, tuning into each other. The combination of her mother's touch, prosody and rhythmic movement calms the neural circuits that have been triggered by Sally's primal stress response (fear and panic) to feeling unattached and unmet. Tuned into each other, Sally experiences relaxation because her mother is relaxed. She is able to roll soft balls back and forth to me and catch and return balloons, while sitting in her mother's lap.

These props are useful for interaction and empathic response, playfully matching Sally's quality of interaction. For example, if she rolls the ball gently, I roll it back in the same way and encourage her mother to do the same. If she hits a balloon hard, I return it, exactly matching her power and affect, so as to meet with her, but not overwhelm her. By the third session, she also enjoys throwing and catching all the balloons from a cloth the three of us hold. By the fourth session, she directs and maintains the play between the three of us, pumping up a big gym ball, physically separating herself from her mum and, lying back on the sofa, using her legs and feet to push the ball back and forth between us, insisting we take off our shoes and socks and use our feet like her. She delights in her body's energetic and purposeful push and pull.

Over the next few sessions, I introduce soft clay, which she enjoys squishing; wooden blocks, which she balances with exquisite control; animal figures, which she briefly animates on her mother's hands; and soft toys and natural loose parts, which she piles together chaotically.

Although she is 3 years old, Sally's play during these sessions is typical of children aged about 18–20 months. She is curious and exploratory and interested in how the environment responds to her actions. She has a short attention span, and her language reflects random connections between the present moment and recently felt sense experiences. She begins to engage in pretend play for short periods. Thus, in the early stages of a dyadic play therapy intervention, the child has regressed to the security of a developmental stage previous to her traumatic experience of being taken into hiding from her father and leaving the safety and familiarity of her family home.

Through prosody, rhythmic movement and sensitive touch, Tracey re-establishes attunement with Sally, helping them both to settle down and feel safe with each other in the calm presence of the therapist and the safety of the playroom. Through simple, repetitive play experiences, mother and child repattern and modulate their stress responses in playful relationship with the therapist.

## *Charlie, aged 10 years*

Charlie's mother, who has learning disabilities, was unaware of her pregnancy until the third trimester, and then Charlie was taken from her at a few days old because of concerns for his safety. He was placed with a family member. He stayed with them until he was 8 years old and, unfortunately, during this time he witnessed domestic violence and sexual assault and experienced neglect and emotional abuse, with a high probability of physical assault and suspected sexual abuse. He was removed and placed with foster carers. At 8 years old, he was unable to wash and dress himself and was illiterate. His foster mother embarked on caring for him and preparing him for school. In her care, he made swift progress, but, 2 years later, he was referred to play therapy because of his increasingly challenging behaviour, abusive language and emotional meltdowns.

Perry (2004) describes how neural development is sequential. When brainstem and midbrain development is disrupted through neglect and trauma, the infant will not have experienced appropriate protection and core emotional regulation with an attuned carer. With no one to regulate him, he will be unregulated all the time, never experiencing rest and calm and utterly unable to manage by himself the overwhelming fear and panic induced by a chaotic environment. Subsequent development in the limbic and cortical domains will be dominated by chronic stress, manifesting in Charlie's case as hypervigilance, defiance and aggression, overriding the developing social engagement system and keeping the child in a perpetual state of reactivity to perceived threat, even when the real threat has been removed.

Intervention included:

- the therapeutic touchstone story (Prendiville, 2014b) in the presence of the child and his carer; the therapist succinctly and in an age-appropriate way tells the child his story through play figures, to let the child know what the therapist knows about him, to establish transparency and safety, and to pave the way for the child to retell it, in his own time, in his own way;
- non-intrusive responding, reflection and tracking, supporting the child's therapeutic experience of core regulation;
- spontaneous therapeutic interventions to calm and soothe the child's dysregulation through initiating echo, mimicry and mirroring play – for example: humming, singing, squishing soft clay and hand washing;
- psycho-education for the foster carer regarding attachment and co-regulation of hyperaroused states.

In Session 7, unpredictable rule-based play reflects Charlie's confusion and his attempts to control the world. He sets up a complicated sequence of tasks for me to complete, with a scoring system. I follow his instructions closely, and he gives orders, unpredictably changing his instructions while getting quite cross with me. I feel slow and stupid, and I verbalize how confused I feel, aware that, if I am right, I am reflecting back to Charlie what it is like to be him. He relaxes and laughs, which tells me I may be on the right track. He then decides we are to swap roles. He does the course himself, and I have to tell him when he is to change task. I do this calmly and carefully, being consistent and making sure he has time to pay attention to what he is doing. I am taking great care of him.

He explains rules for a game of 'music and dance' – when his drumming stops, I must stop dancing. I keep my attention on him and reflect back how hard it is to keep up with the sudden changes in rhythm. I am aware that, again, I am feeling what it is like to be Charlie. He enjoys playing the drum and gradually becomes entranced by it. Then he tells me to play the drum, and he dances, rhythmically and unselfconsciously. It feels like a release, and I feel very joyful. I keep playing, and he stops, breathless, and then says 'Faster!', dancing again, brilliantly and wildly. He picks up a soft blanket and drapes it over his head and continues to dance. He tells me to drape the blanket over both of us, as we must dance together. The blanket encloses us both in one single shadowed space that shuts out the world outside. He then twists himself into the blanket and falls back against me, telling me to hold him. Falling backwards demands unconditional trust, and he shows me that he feels safe with my arms wrapped around him in the soft blanket. He then tells me to do the same with him (to fall backwards into his arms), but I say that I am big and he is small, and it is my job to keep us safe. He accepts this and repeats the same movement a few more times, with the blanket wrapped tightly around his body and over his head.

At a physiological level, he is looking for trust, acceptance and feedback from his environment. In therapeutic relationship, he demonstrates his primal need to be caught and held, for caring touch, pressure and positive feedback from the world. Gil (2010) believes that, in therapy, the processes that children find on their own are equal to, or often surpass, the solutions that their therapists may propose: 'Clinical interventions that allow children to find their own way towards healing may prove to be extremely helpful and child-friendly' (p. 10).

## Ben, aged 13 years

Ben was referred because of his parents' difficult separation and his mother's concerns for his well-being. Both his parents gave consent for therapy. Ben is dyslexic. He gets very stressed before learning situations. He shuts down, his parasympathetic nervous system activated in a defensive, dissociated state. In educational psychological assessment, he has been described as autistic and unteachable. During intake, his mother tells me that she had initiated the separation from Ben's father 6 months before and his father refused to believe it, actively resisting her wishes and very reluctant to move out of the house. This had caused great distress for the children. Ben's father is particularly attached to Ben and, according to Ben's mother, he actively encourages symbiosis, identifying with Ben's problems as his own and projecting his own experience of the world on to Ben, who is his eldest son. As Ben enters adolescence, he is struggling to define himself as separate from his father.

Intervention focused on:

- outdoor therapeutic play sessions;
- identifying and working with boundary themes that emerged in his play;
- therapeutic use of self, particularly in approach behaviour and embodied listening;
- staying within the metaphor of the play;
- providing support and psycho-education to his mother regarding co-regulation of hypoarousal, particularly dissociation.

Themes of boundaries emerge every session, working from outside inwards. Ben makes a 'guardian of the wood' from found natural objects, to stand guard at the entrance to the wood. On another occasion, he constructs stone cairns to mark the pathway into the wood. I encourage him to define personal (kinaesthetic) space and to imagine a boundary that keeps out what is not wanted. He draws a personal boundary on the ground with a stick and imagines what it is made of. Then he collects found objects from the woodland floor to symbolize what he wants to keep inside his boundary.

During fire-making, Ben shows awareness of skin as a boundary. He remarks that he can feel the heat of the fire on his leg and he imagines keeping a monster away with a boundary of fire. He makes the monster from mud and sticks and places it out beyond the boundary of the woodland site.

He engages in activities exploring touch, smell, taste and sensing time passing. During one such session, Ben closes his eyes, counting by feel some acorns placed in the palm of his hand. He enjoys roasting and tasting them and comparing their shape and taste with hazelnuts. He searches for just the right word to describe each different taste. Rather than letting me keep time by checking my watch, Ben prefers to guess how much time has passed.

Gradually overcoming his fear of leaving the ground, he balances on a slack rope, climbs a tree and lies quietly in the hammock. He tunes in to proprioception – his inner sense of where his body is in space and in relation to ground and how he is moving (Ayres, 2005; Frank and La Barre, 2011). During this process, he begins sensing inner sensations of difficult emotions and, with support, he practises moving through them: he gets frustrated and annoyed; he has a bad headache; feeling nauseous, he stomps around the fire; he finds his voice, calling out and swearing; and, finally, he douses the fire with a whole bucket of water. Expressing his frustration liberates his body, shifting him from a toxic, frozen, hurting state into fluid, joyful movement.

During the following sessions, he becomes absorbed in messy, sensory, immersive play. He melts wax in a pot on the fire and mixes it with ash, soil and leaves. Manipulating the soft, warm wax with his fingers and dipping his whole hand in, he peels it off, immersed in what that feels like.

Engaging with natural materials and the elements, Ben developed a stronger sense of himself in relationship with the therapist and his environment. From being without boundaries in the world, he was able to begin to differentiate exteroception (noticing how he receives and responds to sensory information from the environment) from interoception (his ability to notice how he feels, moves and senses within his body). As he did this, he was able to communicate his experiences and, by naming them, own them. He was better able to stay present and dissociated less often. He began to sustain engagement with people, making friends and, on occasions, questioning rules and testing boundaries. He was referred for specialist help with his dyslexia.

Ben has made extraordinary progress in all domains. He found a sense of self, by defining first his outermost boundary and proceeding inwards, finding his way back in time to his earliest-felt sense memories of being in the world through his 'tactile–kinesthetic body' (Sheets-Johnstone, 1998: 275).

## *Alice, aged 39 years*

Alice's intake session included making a family constellation. At the centre of it, she placed her mother, defensive and hyperactive, working herself into exhaustion managing everything. Alice's father has a history of depression, but her mother managed him too, reducing the impact of his illness on the children. Alice remembers a happy early childhood. However, a family friend sexually abused both her and her younger sister, when she was 9 years old and her sister was 6. He was babysitting them. Her parents moved the family away, and she forgot about it until she saw him again when she was 16 and had a vivid flashback memory of the abuse. She told her mother and her sister, hoping for him to be reported, but nothing happened except that the man was gradually and permanently excluded from the extended family. Apart from that, he remains unpunished. To this day, Alice feels her mother's doubt, and her sister denies the abuse. Alice has been living with the feeling of abandonment and not being believed ever since. As a teenager, she was hospitalized for short periods. She experiences debilitating autonomic reactions (shaking and mild fits) to sensory stimulus, particularly noise. She has a history of self-medication and seeking help through different therapies. She is highly verbal, working hard to understand and make sense of her memories and flashbacks in terms of patterns and symmetries. She describes an avalanche of different feelings that accompany these thought processes. Secrets and silence around the abuse have resulted in her feelings of being unsupported, responsible and angry. As an adult, these feelings surface in other, unrelated, contexts, particularly resulting from perceived misunderstandings and misinformation in her professional life.

Intervention focused on:

- establishing the therapeutic relationship between the client, the therapist and the environment, supporting regulation and facilitating self-expression;
- finding memories of a safe place;
- listening with the body, tracking the client's thought processes and reflecting feelings;
- the therapist monitoring her own responses very carefully and modulating her responses;
- psycho-education about autonomic reactivity, attachment and regulation;
- witnessing the client moving in nature: 'being seen' empathically.

*Session 1*

We go to the stream, and I give her a selection of stones to immerse in the water and to arrange as she likes. The stones look grey when they are dry but glow in fantastic colours and patterns when wet. She notices and enjoys their transformation. Then she begins to cry. She is remembering freezing in front of her peers. I sense the need for a 'brake', as her energy is escalating. I guide her back to the stones and the water. She calms down with her hands in the stream. I get out the clay and suggest she collects things from the woods and makes a creature. She stands and begins to collect things. I feel she is still agitated. I pay close attention to her, tracking my own feelings out loud, and she comes over to where I am by the stream. I offer her some clay, holding the same amount in my hand. I then closely mirror her movements with the clay, tracking how it feels to be rolling it with my thumb, the weight of it, the texture, the temperature.

She says, 'I cant think what to make.'

I say, 'You can't think what to make but your fingers seem to know exactly what they are doing.'

Thus, gradually, she becomes curious about what she is making, and then she begins to make decisions about it, immersing herself in imaginary play. When she finishes, I suggest she finds a safe place for her clay figure. She finds a hole at the base of a tree. She puts the clay figure there, looking out, but hidden by a stick and fern leaves. She smiles, satisfied.

*Session 2*

I explain the need for resourcing and its power to regulate; how, at times of overwhelm, finding a memory of a safe place can bring feelings of warmth and care, and slow down the heart beat and rate of breathing, calming the aroused autonomic nervous system (Rothschild, 2000).

Alice chooses clay. She shapes the clay as she speaks about memories of her first home. This triggers a journey through sadness: being moved from that beloved house. She finds it hard to breathe. I suggest she moves. At first, all she can do is move her fingers on the clay. Then she moves her body, and her breathing deepens. She cries with the release.

I ask her, 'What is going on for you?'

She says, 'I need to curl up.'

I make a nest of soft blankets and cushions, and she curls up. She speaks of a memory of curling up in the giant laundry basket, as a very young child. It feels warm and safe. It is an embodied memory, and she smiles and relaxes for a while, enjoying the soft blankets. When she sits up, I hand her the clay shape she made, which she holds and says is a space for a small child to curl up in, like a walnut shell. She keeps it as a symbol of her first 'safe place' memory.

For many adults, the abstract, thinking mind, located in the left-brain tertiary cortex and not fully developed until our mid 20s, can generate thought patterns that, as a defence mechanism, shut off re-experiencing painful embodied memories of childhood trauma. Alice trained as a professional dancer and she also has highly developed and conscious control of her movement repertoire. She was, in a sense, doubly defended, bound by her coping strategies and her training. Therapeutic intervention focused, primarily and over several sessions, on establishing resources for safety, establishing trust and regulating brainstem and midbrain using sensory play, spontaneous movement and expressive arts, usually followed by 10 minutes of free movement in nature, silently witnessed by the therapist, at the end of each session. Although this was just a beginning, Alice reports that she feels the benefit of the resources she found during the ten sessions, noticing that she is better able to look after herself and feels more resilient.

## Conclusion

We have brought together evidence to show that the nervous system develops in a continuum of environmental interaction, from conception, through the birthing process, then, as a newborn, yielding to the arms and gaze of the mother, and onwards in relationship, through developmental stages across the lifespan: an ongoing process of millions of repeated experiences that consolidate synaptic connections, associating movement, touch, sensory perception and primary emotions.

Analysis asks for differentiation between body systems, but, in reality, reflecting on the origins of life, every system has achieved its state of development in cooperation and partnership with other bodily systems and in environmental relationship. The development of the whole person is shaped by this history. The aim of this chapter is to guide practitioners to search for integrated understanding of the whole person's reality in the present moment. To an aware practitioner, our past is always detectable in the present.

The case studies show how, in play therapy and creative psychotherapy, children, adolescents and adults will find their own way back to a time when they felt safe and at one with the world and, from there, with the support of an empathic, synchronous and attuned therapeutic relationship, using movement, prosody and touch, they begin the work of reconstructing the narrative of their lives, making sense, connecting with and integrating what has happened to them.

## Key points

- In human development, movement and touch underpin all the other senses.
- Our earliest experiences of movement and touch leave an imprint on the way we engage in relationships and environmental interactions, from early attachment and throughout our lives.
- Safety, predictability and nurturance are the key principles of core regulation and can be established in therapeutic relationship through prosody and playful movement and touch experiences.

## References

Ayres, J.A. (2005). *Sensory Integration and the Child: Understanding hidden sensory challenges* (25th Anniversary edn). Los Angeles, CA: Western Psychological Services.

Bainbridge Cohen, B. (2012). *Sensing, Feeling, and Action: The experiential anatomy of body–mind centering* (3rd edn). Northampton, MA: Contact Editions.

Booth, P.B., and Jernberg, A.M. (2010). *Theraplay: Helping parents and children build better relationships through attachment-based play* (3rd edn). San Francisco, CA: John Wiley.

Brook, A. (2001). *From Conception to Crawling: Foundations for developmental movement.* Body-Mind.NET.

Brown, S. (2009). *Play: How it shapes the brain, opens the imagination and invigorates the soul.* New York: Avery.

Cattanach, A. (1994). *Play Therapy: Where the sky meets the underworld.* London: Jessica Kingsley.

Dykema, R. (2006). How your nervous system sabotages your ability to relate. An interview with Stephen Porges about his polyvagal theory. Available at: http://stephenporges.com/index.php/component/content/article/5-popular-articles/18-an-interview-with-stephen-porges-about-his-polyvagal-theory (accessed 26 May 2016).

Fearn, M. (2015). Notes from a case study (unpublished).
Feldman, R. (2007). Parent–infant synchrony and the construction of shared timing: Physiological precursors, developmental outcomes and risk conditions. *Journal of Child Psychology and Psychiatry*, *48*(3/4), 329–54.
Frank, R., and La Barre, F. (2011). *The First Year and the Rest of your Life: Movement, development and psychotherapeutic change*. New York: Routledge.
Gallese, V. (2007). Before and below 'theory of mind': Embodied simulation and the neural correlates of social cognition. *Philosophical Transactions of the Royal Society*, *B362*, 659–69.
Gerhardt, S. (2005). *Why Love Matters: How affection shapes a baby's brain*. Hove, UK: Routledge.
Gil, E. (2010) *Working with Children to Heal Interpersonal Trauma: The power of play*. New York: Guilford Press.
Grof, S., and Bennett, H.Z. (1992). *The Holotropic Mind: The three levels of human consciousness and how they shape our lives*. San Francisco, CA: Harper Collins.
Harlow, H.F., and Zimmermann, R.R. (1959). Affectional responses in the infant monkey. *Science*, 130(Aug), 421–32.
Jennings, S. (1999). *Introduction to Developmental Playtherapy*. London: Jessica Kingsley.
Jennings, S. (2011). *Healthy Attachments and Neuro-Dramatic-Play*. London: Jessica Kingsley.
Levine, P.A., and Kline, M. (2007). *Trauma Through a Child's Eyes: Awakening the ordinary miracle of healing; infancy through adolescence*. Berkley, CA: North Atlantic Books.
McCarty, M. (2014). *Is there a relationship between children's birth experiences and their conceptualisation of a safe place?* Unpublished dissertation for MA in Humanistic and Integrative Play Therapy, CTC, Eire.
Montagu, A. (1978). *Touching: The human significance of the skin*. New York: Harper & Row.
Norton, C.C., and Norton, B.E. (2008). Experiential play therapy. In C.E. Schaefer and H.G. Kaduson (eds) *Contemporary Play Therapy: Theory, research and practice* (pp. 28–54). New York: Guilford Press.
Panksepp, J., and Biven, L. (2012). *The Archaeology of Mind*. New York: Norton.
Perry, B.D. (2000). *The Neuroarchaeology of Childhood Maltreatment: The neuro-developmental costs of adverse childhood events*. The Child Trauma Academy. Available at: www.juconicomparte.org/recursos/Neuroarcheology%20of%20childhood%20maltreatment_zmH8.pdf (accessed 30 May 2016).
Perry, B.D. (2004). Violence and childhood. In Perry, B.D. (2004) *Understanding Traumatized and Maltreated Children: The core concepts* [DVD]. Houston, TX: The Child Trauma Academy.
Perry, B.D. (2008). Child maltreatment: A neurodevelopmental perspective on the role of abuse in psychopathology. In T.P. Beauchaine and S.P. Hinshaw (eds) *Child and Adolescent Psychopathology* (pp. 93–128). New York: Wiley.
Perry, B.D., and Hambrick, E.P (2008). The neurosequential model of therapeutics. *Reclaiming Children and Youth*, *17*(3), 38–43.
Perry, B.D, and Szalavitz, M. (2006). *The Boy Who Was Raised as a Dog, and Other Stories from a Child Psychiatrist's Notebook*. New York: Basic Books.

Porges, S.W. (2003). The polyvagal theory: Phylogenetic contributions to social behavior. *Physiology & Behavior, 79*, 503–13.
Porges, S.W. (2011). 'Somatic perspectives' series: Interview with Serge Prengel. USABP and EABP. Available at: www.SomaticPerspectives.com (accessed 16 May 2016).
Prasad, N. (2011). *Using a Neurodevelopmental Lens when Working with Children Who Have Experienced Maltreatment: A review of the literature of Bruce D. Perry*. NSW: UnitingCare.
Prendiville, E. (2014a). Abreaction. In C.E. Schaefer and A.A. Drewes (eds) *The Therapeutic Powers of Play: 20 core agents of change* (2nd edn; pp. 83–109). New York: Wiley.
Prendiville, E. (2014b). The therapeutic touchstone. In E. Prendiville and J. Howard (eds) *Play Therapy Today: Contemporary practice with individuals, groups and carers* (pp. 7–28). Abingdon, UK: Routledge.
Rank, O. (1993). *The Trauma of Birth*. New York: Dover.
Rizzolatti, G., Fogassi, L., and Gallese, V. (2006). Mirrors in the mind. *Scientific American, 295*, 54–61.
Rothschild, B. (2000). *The Body Remembers: The psychophysiology of trauma and trauma treatment*. New York: W.W. Norton.
Sampaio, R.C., and Truwit, C.L. (2001). Myelination in the developing human brain. In *Handbook of Developmental Cognitive Neuroscience* (pp. 35–44). Cambridge, MA: MIT Press.
Schaefer, C.E., and Drewes, A.A. (2014). *The Therapeutic Powers of Play: 20 core agents of change* (2nd edn). New York: Wiley.
Schoenwolf, G.C., Bleyl, S.B., Brauer, P.R., and Francis-West, P.H. (2009). *Larsen's Human Embryology* (4th edn). Philadelphis, PA: Churchill Livingstone-Elsevier.
Schore, A.N. (2002). The neurobiology of attachment and early personality organisation. *Journal of Prenatal & Perinatal Psychology & Health, 16*(3), 249–63.
Schore, A.N. (2005). Back to basics: Attachment, affect regulation, and the developing right brain: linking developmental neuroscience to paediatrics. *Paediatrics in Review, 26*(6), 204–17.
Schore, A.N. (2011). The right brain implicit self lies at the core of psychoanalysis. *Psychoanalytic Dialogues, 21*, 75–100.
Sheets-Johnstone, M. (1998). Consciousness: A natural history. *Journal of Consciousness Studies, 5*(3), 260–94.
Siegel, D.J. (2012). *The Developing Mind: How relationships and the brain interact to shape who we are*. New York: Guilford Press.
Sori, C.F., and Schnur, S. (2013). Integrating a neurosequential approach to the treatment of traumatized children: An interview with Eliana Gil, Part II. *The Family Journal: Counseling & Therapy for Couples & Families*. DOI: 10.1177/1066 480713514945.
Stagnitti, K. (2009). Play intervention – The learn to play program. In K. Stagnitti and R. Cooper (eds) *Play as Therapy* (pp. 178–86). London: Jessica Kingsley.
Stamenov, N.I., and Gallese, V. (2002). *Mirror Neurons and the Evolution of Brain and Language*. Amsterdam: John Benjamins.
Stern, D.N. (1985). *The Interpersonal World of the Infant: A view from psychoanalysis and Developmental Psychology*. New York: Basic Books.

Sunderland, M. (2006). *The Science of Parenting*. London: Dorling Kindersley.
Vinnikov, Y.A. (1974). *Sensory Reception: Cytology, molecular mechanisms and evolution* (trans. W.L. Gray and B. Crook). Molecular Biology, Biochemistry and Biophysics series, vol. 17. Berlin: Springer-Verlag.
Whelan, W.F. and Stewart, A.L. (2014). Attachment. In C.E. Schaefer and A.A. Drewes (eds) *The Therapeutic Powers of Play: 20 core agents of change* (2nd edn, pp. 171–83). Hoboken, NJ: Wiley.
Yasenik, L., and Gardner, K. (2012). *Play Therapy Dimensions Model: A decision making guide for integrative play therapists*. London: Jessica Kingsley.

Chapter 7

# Coming alive
Finding joy through sensory play

*Siobhán Prendiville and Maggie Fearn*

## Introduction

This chapter will provide an introduction to sensory play, explain its potential benefits for all ages and stages of development, and include neurobiological theory that underpins a developmental approach for using sensory play in play therapy. Case study examples across the lifespan bring to life the extraordinary power of sensory play for healing chronic nervous system reactivity to stress and trauma.

Essentially, sensory play engages the child and stimulates or soothes the nervous system, helping with organization, integration and regulation. Ayres clarifies that, 'parents may not realise that their child's learning and behaviour problems are the result of neurological disorders that the child cannot control' (2005: 51). Sensory play provides children, adolescents and adults with the opportunity to perceive their internal and external environments and to process sensory information and make sense of what is going on. Sensory memories are retained only briefly; most are discarded within milliseconds. However, if linked with attention and emotion (the pleasure of play), the sensory memory can pass into short-term memory and, with repetition, into long-term memory, making synaptic connections and developing neural pathways in the brain and stimulating corticol development (Perry *et al.*, 2000).

Our five external senses are commonly known as tactile sense (touch), olfactory sense (smell), gustatory sense (taste), auditory sense (hearing) and visual sense (sight) (Beckerleg, 2009: 48). If we consider the senses as the mode by which the body communicates both external and internal stimuli to and from the brain, then there are at least three more inner senses or sensory systems linked to proprioception – the sensing of our own movements (Frank, 2001; Godwin Emmons and McKendry Anderson, 2005; Gascoyne, 2012). From infancy to adulthood, proprioception encompasses all movement and includes integration of:

- kinaesthetic awareness, which is our sense of weight, action or stillness, resistance, and relative positioning in relationship with the environment;
- vestibular awareness, which is spatial awareness, awareness of direction of motion in space and relative positioning of the body in relationship with gravity;

- visceral awareness, which is sensitivity to pulsations of organs giving information about energy levels and fatigue (Frank, 2001).

By combining proprioceptive awareness with our external sensing, we are able to orientate ourselves and respond towards or away from sensory information. Neurons associated with the proprioceptive sense are located within the ear, muscles, tendons and joints and connect via the spinal cord to the somatosensory cortex (Frank, 2001; Godwin Emmons and McKendry Anderson, 2005; Gascoyne, 2012). The inner, middle and outer ears coordinate balance and hearing and work together with the visual system. Sight is one of the more underdeveloped senses at birth (Gascoyne, 2012).

The skin, the largest organ of the human body, is the sensory organ responsible for touch. Varying types of touch receptor located within the layers of skin identify and register pressure, light touch, pain, heat and cold. These touch receptors are unevenly dispersed across the body, with the bulk of them located in the hands, lips, genitals and mouth. Sensing through movement, touch, hearing and smell is developed *in utero*. Although the neural systems for smell and taste are distinct from each other, they are inextricably linked and often work together. The olfactory bulb and tract, the area of the brain with responsibility for evaluating and relaying smells, is positioned in the limbic region of the brain, close to the hippocampus, the area of the brain that holds particular significance in forming memories and connecting emotions and senses to memories (Gascoyne, 2012). Taste receptors are positioned on the tongue, roof of the mouth and inside the cheeks. Babies begin to develop their sense of taste while still *in utero*, swallowing the amniotic fluid (Beckerleg, 2009). It is proposed that frequently reoccurring tastes experienced in the womb become registered in a baby's memory (Gascoyne, 2012). Although taste receptors identify sweet, sour, salty and bitter tastes, smell, touch and texture also significantly impact upon the entire taste sensation.

## Sensory play and sensory integration

For the purpose of explaining the senses, they have been differentiated; however, they interact and work together with all the body systems. Sensory play experiences generally provide a multi-systemic context for the exploration and development of a range of experiences promoting and fostering sensory, affective and regulatory integration. Such experiences develop a child's capacity 'to feel, understand, and organize sensory information from his body and his environment' and are fundamental to homeostasis, growth and development (Godwin Emmons and McKendry Anderson, 2005: 14). According to Fearn (2014), through engaging in sensory play, the child can develop 'the ability to receive sensory information, regulate and manage incoming sensations and respond within a comfortable range of arousal' (p. 114). Gerhardt (2004) highlights the relationship between sensation, perception and regulation in the attachment relationship, the mother's process internalized and integrated by the child via attunement and co-regulation. In developing her sensory attachment interventions for treating children who have suffered trauma or neglect, Eadaoin Breathneach trains occupational therapists to focus on identifying each child's particular reactive style of sensory relatedness and then instigates a sensory programme that changes daily living routines in order to calm, soothe and adjust the child's nervous system and support the development of self-regulation (West, 2011).

## Sensory play and child development

The work of Piaget (1896–1980) is critical in the development and understanding of sensory play and its contribution to child development, particularly the foundations of emerging cognitive development. Cortical brain development during the first 7 years is profoundly influenced by and integrated through sensory experience. Huttenlocher (2002) describes an early period of rapid growth, from birth to 2 years, establishing the basic functions of the different cortical regions, and the period from 1 year old to early adolescence is characterized by 'exuberant connections' in the cerebral cortex (p. 80), which correlates with heightened plasticity in response to environmental stimulation. Piaget proposes that children's sensory engagement and interactions with the environment create learning possibilities and enable them to build up direct knowledge of the world. He describes the earliest stage in a child's development as the sensorimotor stage, whereby the majority of a child's learning during their first 2 years occurs through the senses (Piaget, 1954, 1964). He proposes that babies and toddlers need to move, manipulate and explore a variety of objects, in order to initially develop an understanding of their qualities, and later progress to an understanding of object permanence – the knowledge that objects continue to exist even when they can no longer be seen, a vital step in the development of imagination and thinking skills.

The cortex develops via input from the sense organs and other key cortical areas, forming functionary circuits and becoming stabilized (Huttenlocher, 2002). Through exploratory play activities such as balancing, sitting, reaching, grasping, holding and releasing, children develop their ability to control and coordinate their bodies. The self-led, open-ended component of such play enables children to explore their sensory preferences and contributes to their developing sense of self, identity and confidence, while simultaneously providing opportunities to communicate and express themselves, either verbally or nonverbally. The move into symbolic thought, when toddlers begin forming mental representations of the play objects and using mental predictions and planning while playing with the materials, also supports linguistic development, as children begin to use symbols and sounds to communicate (Williamson and Anzalone, 1997; Tassoni and Hucker, 2005; Beckerleg, 2009; Jennings, 2011; Gascoyne, 2012; Gaskill, 2014; Prendiville, 2014).

## Sensory play and play development

Sensory-rich play experiences are critical in children's play development (Stagnitti, 1998, 2009; Jennings, 1999). According to Stagnitti (1998), children need to engage in sensory and exploratory play with objects before they can progress on to more complex imaginative, pretend play. Typically, during the second year of life, the predominant sensory play involving manipulation and exploration gives way to pretend play (Pulaski, 1976; Stagnitti, 1998). Pretend play initially develops when young children imitate adults and other children. It is a complex form of play that requires the child to have mastered a number of foundation skills associated with regular sensory play experiences, such as: movement, sensory integration, manipulation, object permanency, imitation and relating objects (McCune-Nicolich, 1977; Stagnitti, 1998).

Sensory play involves the moving body. Jennings (1999) calls this type of play 'embodiment play'. Embodiment is the first of three stages Jennings outlines in her developmental paradigm, Embodiment–Projection–Role (EPR), which, along with neuro-dramatic play (Jennings, 2011), charts the progression of dramatic play from birth to 7 years. Children engage in physical play, including, for example rhythmic movement, clapping games and rough-and-tumble play. These activities stimulate the lower regions of the brain (Perry, 2006). Jennings (2014) proposes that such activities are crucial in the development of body self and body image. A child's embodied development can be disrupted or distorted for many reasons, including hospitalization, early life trauma, neglect and play deprivation. If early developmental disruption occurs, it is necessary to provide ample opportunities for movement play, regardless of chronological age.

## Sensory play and environment

The outdoors provides a multitude of sensory-rich experiences that encourage and promote absorption in movement and sensory play. Jumping in a muddy puddle, rolling down a hill, climbing in a sand dune, digging in soil, feeling the heat of the sun as it hits your neck or the coolness of the rain as it brushes against your cheek, smelling flowers or indeed cow dung, crawling or running through long swishy grass, tasting fresh berries plucked from the plant or walking and exploring in the forest, the outdoors offers limitless, multilayered, sensory-rich play experiences made up of sights, sounds, feelings, textures, smells, tastes and opportunities to explore movement. Fearn (2014) explores the importance of incorporating the natural environment as 'a significant presence in the therapeutic relationship and as a fundamental pre-requisite for integrated sensory-motor development' (p. 113).

A well-planned indoor environment can also provide sensory-rich play experiences for children, adolescents and adults. This can include providing resources to encourage whole-body movement, such as tents, tunnels, large gym balls, sponge balls, cloths of different textures and colours, soft cushions and blankets; the sense of space can change with different lighting options; it may involve using natural materials, bringing the outdoors in, and providing accessible containers of a wide range of different sensory play resources.

The environment shapes neurobiological development throughout the lifespan, with the majority of brain organization occurring in the first 4 years (Huttenlocher, 2002; Perry, 2006; Panksepp and Biven, 2012). A sensory play environment needs to provide rich, diverse sensory immersion that attunes and engages the whole child through movement, touch, sight, sounds and smells in a preconscious process of sensation–perception–integration that stimulates right-brain growth, providing the sensory, regulatory, creative, nonverbal, preconscious background that informs socio-emotional development (Cozolino, 2010; Porges, 2011). Our perception of safety is formed in the experiential right brain from our earliest environmental experiences. Memories are often recalled as sensory experience and emerge in association with cues from the present. If these stored implicit memories recall a safe, nurturing, richly sensory environment, the child has an inner resource that provides a template for subsequent experiences. If these felt-sense memories are of unsafe, frightening, stressful experiences, therapeutic intervention using sensory-based play can support the child to re-imagine and repattern maladaptive responses that occur in response to implicit memory. As well as establishing a sense of containment and safety in therapeutic relationship, paying attention to the therapeutic play space as an interactive sensory environment facilitates the child's ability to maintain a comfortable range of arousal in brainstem and limbic regions of the brain.

## Neurosequential development and sensory activity

Sensory exploration can be used successfully with all ages, from infants to adults. Perry's neurosequential model of therapeutics (2006) emphasizes the critical need to sequence interventions, activities and experiences in a way that replicates the hierarchical development of the brain and fits with the client's current stage of neurodevelopment, regardless of chronological age. Because of the sequential and hierarchical development of the brain and nervous system, each developmental stage is dependent on the previous stage being successfully negotiated and prefigures the next stage. Without core state regulation being established in the child's inner world through early attachment relationship play, primarily through prosody, movement and touch experiences, the child will not be able to explore the outer world through their senses. Integrating sensory experiences, as well as developing the neural mapping necessary to begin to recognize, differentiate and define those experiences, contributes to the child's emergent sense of self in relationship (Stern, 1985). These experiences consolidate synaptic connections within the limbic area, developing the child's ability to respond and relate to familiar significant others in her immediate environment and prefiguring the next projective, relational stage in her socio-emotional development.

If a child suffers developmental trauma or neglect during the sensorimotor stage, this will impact on their subsequent ability to self-regulate and to be able to relate to the outside world and their ability to integrate and learn from their experiences. Because of environment-dependent neural plasticity, however, that child can have the opportunity to revisit developmental stages at any time during their lifespan and, through appropriate play experiences repeated over time with a developmentally aware play therapist, repattern their nervous system and make up for lost time (Perry, 2006).

According to Bruce (2011), repetitive and patterned rhythmic and sensory-based activities are required to activate and provide organizing neural input to the lower regions of the brain – the brainstem and the midbrain. A child who is lethargic and unresponsive, caught in a parasympathetic state of hypoarousal, needs playful stimulation of the sympathetic nervous system to bring them to calm alertness. Play with sensory materials can also facilitate stress reduction (Bemis, 2014) and be extremely calming and regulating. Dysregulation is a physiological event (Perry, 2006). The lower region of the brain controls the regulatory system. If the brainstem is activated, children, adolescents and adults will experience symptoms such as a change in heart rate and body temperature, altered breathing and poor control over motor functioning. Hyperactive and acting-out behaviours are also associated with activation of the brainstem (Gil, 2013). When dysregulation occurs, the cortex goes 'off line' (Gil, 2013: 2), and, for the person to be able to engage cognitively, the regulatory system must be calmed down or woken up. Play and exploration of sensory materials and creative arts are appropriate for calming and stimulating the nervous system, as are somatosensory activities such as rhythmic movement, rocking, singing, drumming, massage, therapeutic touch and movement, as explored in the previous chapter (Perry, 2006).

## Approaches and resources for sensory-rich play

### Heuristic play and treasure baskets

Goldschmied coined the term 'heuristic play', meaning discovery play, in the 1980s (Goldschmied and Jackson, 1994). Heuristic play is firmly grounded in young children's natural curiosity and involves offering a young child or group of children a wide range of natural, household and recycled materials for exploration and free play, without any unnecessary adult intervention. This provides children with opportunities to engage in sensory exploration and open-ended play with natural materials, such as, for example, sea-shells, conkers, fir-cones, driftwood, loofahs and pebbles, and also manmade objects, such as ribbons, cardboard tubes, brushes, egg cups, curtain rings and hair rollers.

Heuristic play with babies has the senses and sensory exploration at its core and revolves around the treasure basket (Goldschmied and Jackson, 1994). Babies are presented with a flat-bottomed, low-sided basket of sensory-rich natural and household objects and they are simply allowed to play with and explore the objects in whatever way they wish. Heuristic play with toddlers and young children becomes more complex, as they begin to investigate and experiment with the different ways in which the play objects interact with each other. They will explore the range of physical possibilities of an object, through rolling, stacking, dumping, filling, fitting things inside each other, balancing and manipulating in a host of different ways. They will figure out what can be done with the objects and how they can be used together (Gascoyne, 2012). To facilitate this exploration, provide objects that can be used together, for example boxes and tins with lids, baskets that fit inside one another, small objects to put in jars, stick for banging, etc.

Early development is driven by movement: in a safe and familiar environment, the child will relax, and their curiosity will drive exploration of their surrounding environment. All neural development is use-dependent (Perry, 2006). As a young child reaches towards an object that attracts their attention through its shape, colour, texture – their eyes will focus, taking in all the spatial information they need to organize their response via the somatosensory cortex, and they will grasp the object, pull it towards their mouth and explore its sensory characteristics. They receive specific sensations through sensory receptors in their skin that relay information into the spinal cord, sending information into the limbic brain region, forming perceptions of like/dislike, me/not me and beginning to differentiate sensory qualities through experiential learning. Throughout this process, which is repeated over and over again, millions of synaptic connections are firing in the nervous system, integrating somatosensory and emotional experience and forming patterns and loops that inform future actions and experiences. This process develops the body systems that support large body movements, spatial awareness, eye–hand coordination and fine motor skills that engender sensational feedback from their environment, giving the child an increasing sense of effectiveness and control, supporting their exploratory drive and activating their seeking system (Panksepp and Biven, 2012). Perry *et al.* (2000) define play as a combination of curiosity and pleasure. Because it is pleasurable, the child will repeat the experience: repetition is practice, and with practice comes mastery.

## *Messy play resources*

Expanding sensory play to incorporate a wider range of sensory materials, such as sand, water, rice, lentils, pasta, paint, clay, dough, beads, lotions and creams, musical instruments, foods for tasting, ice-cubes, sensory balls and squidgy toys, increases not only the play possibilities but also the benefits associated with the play. Some clients will be drawn to the messy play materials, whereas others may, at least initially, prefer the drier, cleaner play materials.

Providing opportunities for children, adolescents and adults to play with and explore the colours, textures, tastes, smells and sounds of gooey, sticky substances, such as custard, jelly, beans, spaghetti and shaving foam, stimulates their senses and expands sensory awareness in a truly unrestricted fashion. Facilitating experiences to make and play with materials such as play-dough, cloud dough, gloop, cornflour, clay and edible finger paints provides a context for exploring and combining a number of sensory materials.

Art materials, sand, beads, paint and clay provide additional sensory, tactile opportunities in play and are often very successful in engaging older clients, offering a comforting sense of purpose to their play. Providing opportunities for children, adolescents and adults to explore and use such sensory materials in a playful way, at their own pace, without overwhelming them with sensory experiences or forcing them out of their comfort zone, stimulates their senses, promotes sensory integration and enables them to interact more fully with the world around them.

*Relationship enhancement play*

Touch, movement, rhythm and sensory-based play activities are critical components in early developmental and relationship enhancement play. Right-brain to right-brain communication is crucial in emotional regulation and self-regulation and in the development of attachment (Schore, 2005; Schore and Schore, 2008; Cozolino, 2010). Theraplay (Booth and Jernberg, 2010) is a therapeutic intervention based on attachment theory and validated from a neurodevelopmental perspective. Theraplay practitioners direct carer–child dyads in a range of sensory-based activities, such as rocking, feeding, rhythmic movement, singing games and massage, aimed at stimulating this nonverbal, sensory-based region of the brain and promoting positive attachment between parent and child. The stimulation and organization of the lower brain, through somatosensory play-based activities, also work to calm and soothe overactive and hypervigilant children (Munns, 2014).

## Using sensory activities in psychotherapy across the lifespan: Case studies

*Mark, age 7.5 years*

Mark was born to a drug- and alcohol-addicted mother in Eastern Europe, where he spent most of his early years in an orphanage, with a number of failed adoption placements, prior to his adoption and move to Ireland when aged 4. He was referred to play therapy 3 years later as he was experiencing significant sensory, emotional and behavioural difficulties, both at home and in school. These included extremely poor attention skills, atypical motor activity levels, minimal social interactions, significant difficulties in emotional and behavioural regulation, delays in language and cognitive development, severe difficulties falling and staying asleep and very limited awareness of dangers in the environment. In addition, he engaged in self-harming behaviours in the form of pulling his hair out, banging his head repeatedly against the wall, biting his skin from his hands and pulling his nails off.

Initially, Mark's play therapy sessions were non-directive, and he was drawn solely to the sensory materials – sensory balls, squidgy toys, bells, ribbons, boxes, etc. Both his history and his play in the playroom indicated early developmental trauma, and the therapist recognized that he needed an intervention that would make up for lost development, in accordance with the principles of the neuro-sequential model of therapeutics (NMT; Perry, 2006) and neuro-dramatic play (Jennings, 2011). Perry (ibid.) also recommends involving key people in the child's life, so that the play experienced in therapy can be repeated little and often throughout the child's week, repatterning his nervous system. Mark's parents were helped to support him at home: learning playful interaction strategies, incorporating daily sensory and rhythmic play activities, establishing a calm bedtime routine and managing his difficult behaviours in an emotionally sensitive way.

As the play therapy sessions progressed, sensory and messy play resources were provided, in conjunction with early attachment play and rhythmic movement, to stimulate Mark's senses and facilitate the integration of his sensory systems, simultaneously engaging him in relationship-enhancing play through shared experiences, physical contact and co-regulation. Sensory exploration of materials such as sand, water, rice, lentils and pasta predominated in the therapy room, and, later, he played with gloop, play-dough, sand, clay, finger paints, water, lotions, creams and food. Such play proved to be extremely calming for Mark and became a great regulating tool for him in therapy, at home and in school. Treasure basket and heuristic play were introduced both in play therapy sessions and at home.

Developmental movement was explored in playful ways – rolling across the room, crawling through play tunnels, walking on bubble wrap, tumbling in shredded paper and engaging in finger plays, action rhymes and dances such as 'Head, shoulders, knees and toes'. As therapy progressed, he engaged in movement games, body percussion and dance, becoming increasingly aware of what his body could do and how to coordinate his movements.

Work continued with Mark's parents on ways to incorporate such play experiences outside the therapy room. Rough-and-tumble play, sword fighting, play with body movements, outdoor play and baking took place regularly at home. Mark's emerging ability to identify sensations he liked/disliked demonstrated his emerging sense of self and self-identity. Reports from home and school indicated a significant decrease in Mark's emotional outbursts and self-harming behaviours and marked improvements in his relationships with his parents and teachers, attention, motor activity, academic performance, emotional and behavioural regulation and sleep.

As time passed, Mark began to include some symbolic and projective play (Jennings, 1999). The sand he once explored purely on a sensory level became the volcano that erupted and caused chaos for the small world people in the village below; the water was no longer used purely for splashing and feeling: it became the bath water for the baby dolls. Finger paints were used to create images; pasta was used to make necklaces; musical instruments were played during puppet shows; play-dough was turned into people and beings from outer space; the garden became a treasure trove for sensory scavenger hunts, collecting items for sensory tactile collages. Reports from home and school indicated he was now demonstrating an ability to play with peers, take turns, wait, listen to others and share.

He was now identified as having at least one significant friend. Mark continued to move through the EPR stages (Jennings, 1999), and the 'as if', symbolic level of play began to emerge. Dolls, puppets and teddies began to take on roles, as did Mark and his therapist. The bells, leaves, boxes and sticks Mark originally played with to develop his sensory awareness became props for emerging pretend play scenes. The sand and water that had been explored for their sensory qualities now became the desert to be stranded on or the rough sea to sail through to get to safety. At this point, Mark was able to use his pretend play to bring complex thoughts, ideas, feelings and perceptions into focus in his therapy. He was now able to engage in abreactive play (Prendiville, 2014b) and work through and process previously unresolved traumatic memories and experiences.

After 2 years of play therapy, Mark demonstrated significant changes in both his behaviours and development. Mark's teachers and parents reported noticeable improvements in his sensory awareness, emotional and behavioural regulation, play skills, social skills, ability to attend to tasks and work independently, memory recall, academic performance and his general behaviour and mood. Mark displayed appropriate empathy towards other children and now had a number of friends, whom he played with both at home and at school. He regularly used his sensory coping box, which contained play-dough, dry sand, bubbles, hand cream and a squidgy toy. His sleep difficulties had been resolved, he now had a positive, age-appropriate bedtime routine and he no longer engaged in self-harming behaviours.

## *Stephanie, age 15.3 years*

Stephanie had a diagnosis of selective mutism and had been receiving assessment and treatment from various psychologists and speech and language therapists since she was 5 years old. As yet, no treatment had been successful. The only people whom she had ever spoken to were her mother, Mary, and her maternal grandparents. Mary reported that she was concerned about Stephanie's selective mutism and also her 'low moods', 'temper' and emotional 'meltdowns'. She had a strong desire for Stephanie to begin talking and felt that this would help her to identify and manage her feelings. The therapist explained that the therapy would not be a targeted intervention to encourage Stephanie to speak, but rather a psychotherapeutic process using creative media to help Stephanie achieve emotional well-being. In contrast to Mary's belief that Stephanie needed to talk in order to better understand and manage her feelings, the therapist felt it was crucial to help Stephanie gain an understanding of her feelings in order to be able to speak.

Stephanie's therapy process began with the therapeutic touchstone (Prendiville, 2014a). The therapist used this play-based story intervention to present Stephanie with a synopsis of significant elements in her life history. This included details of her life, her relationships, her personality, her emotional outbursts and her selective mutism. It also introduced her to the therapist and creative psychotherapy and clearly stated that it is a space in which clients can speak or not speak.

Stephanie agreed to an initial contract, drawn up using art materials, for twelve sessions of creative psychotherapy.

### The choice bag

In early sessions, Stephanie's anxieties were so intense that she was unable to select any of the creative materials to engage with. A 'choice bag' of possible activities was introduced. Suggestions ranged from exploring the sensory box, painting, finger-painting, clay, sand, making play-dough, creative visualization, story, to talking, playing, listening to music and dancing. Stephanie would pull an idea from the bag and decide whether or not she wanted to do it in that session. This choice bag was used throughout Stephanie's therapy process; as the sessions progressed, both Stephanie and the therapist added new suggestions to the choice bag – for example, hand massage, body percussion and manicure.

During her initial sessions, she explored the sensory materials but remained expressionless, and her body language was extremely rigid. She never spoke or made any sound at all. Even her breathing was exceptionally quiet. The therapist's commentary focused on the sensory qualities of the materials being explored, Stephanie's actions, body language and, occasionally, her quietness. As the sessions progressed, Stephanie began to make eye contact and show basic facial expressions. As the therapist gently responded and wondered about Stephanie's experiences, Stephanie began to expand her nonverbal communications through pointing, gestures, writing and more elaborate facial expressions. She began identifying materials and objects she liked and disliked and gradually widened the repertoire of sensory materials she explored.

### The sensory box

She now included food items such as rice, lentils and pasta, a wide array of sensory balls, scarves, lengths of fabric, musical instruments, bubbles, bubble wrap and moon sand. The therapist suggested that they put together a small sensory box of soothing materials that Stephanie could use at home when she began to feel overwhelmed, angry or worried. Stephanie chose sand, lentils, bubbles, sensory foam and some ribbons for her personal sensory box.

### Messy play

Stephanie began making play-dough, cloud dough and gloop, spending whole sessions simply engaging with the sensory materials and exploring different consistencies. The range and complexity of her facial expressions grew, and her body language became much easier to read and reflect on. Her movements and the sounds she made were becoming less controlled; however, she still did not speak. The therapist's commentary could now focus more on reflecting feelings, rather than simply content.

*The sandtray*

She began exploring the sandtray, initially feeling, raking, sprinkling and moving the sand around, and then adding miniatures to create scenes. When prompted to name her creation, she was unable to do so. She would pick up a marker and place it on a page but simply could not write down a name.

After the twelve initial sessions, Stephanie and her mother reported that Stephanie's general mood was improving at home, she was using the sensory coping box regularly, was experiencing fewer 'meltdowns' and appeared 'lighter' and 'happier going to school'. She spoke to her mother about eventually talking to her friends, but said she was not yet ready. A second contract for ten therapy sessions was agreed.

*Expressive arts*

During the second stage of Stephanie's therapy, she continued to use the choice bag and she began spontaneously exploring more materials in the therapy room and using them to create images, collages, figures and people. She used these creations to share personal details; she began to open up about herself, visually expressing her preferences, her friends and life experiences. She used sensory materials such as feathers, laces, fabric and fibre to create a personal collage, finger paints to do self-portraits and paints and pastels to create preference boards depicting, for example, clothes, music, foods she liked/disliked.

She created people from play-dough and clay to represent her friends and family members. The therapist suggested she develop profiles outlining personality traits, hobbies, likes and dislikes to accompany these characters. Stephanie happily engaged with these, and the therapist made observations, comments and reflections on her work.

Stephanie made salt dough and created imprints of her hands and feet in it. The therapist focused her commentary on how unique and special these prints were. When cooked and set, Stephanie took immense pride in decorating, signing and dating her prints. Although she still did not speak in her therapy sessions, she was communicating extremely effectively.

At this point, Stephanie still did not speak to any adults or peers who were known to her. However, she began to set herself, and achieve, challenges each week – to talk to a shop assistant, to ask a random stranger a question, to speak to a teenager she did not know. Each week, during therapy, she would inform the therapist in writing what she had achieved. Reports from home and school indicated that Stephanie was doing well and appeared happier and more settled. Stephanie's mother reported that, although the frequency and severity of Stephanie's 'meltdowns' had reduced significantly, they still occurred when she became overwhelmed, and she continued to experience difficulties naming her emotions.

Another contract was agreed for ten more sessions of therapy. The therapist named Stephanie's ongoing difficulty recognizing, naming and expressing her feelings, and they agreed to target this in the coming sessions. Stephanie outlined her intent to begin talking to her friends at home, and also in school.

*Using coloured sand, rhythm, sound and creative visualization to explore feelings*

Through the choice bag, the therapist introduced the idea of creating coloured sand and linking this sand to feelings, exploring feelings through music and movement, and using guided imagery and artwork to identify feeling states in the body. Using salt and food colouring, Stephanie created coloured sand and, in turn, created feelings jars. She selected different colours to represent different feeling states and then used these jars to identify feelings associated with both fictional and real-life experiences.

Stephanie then moved into creating sounds using musical instruments and body percussion to accompany the coloured sand. The therapist introduced an activity to identify where Stephanie experienced different feelings in her body. Stephanie lay on a large piece of paper, and the therapist drew an outline of her body. Stephanie then listened to a creative visualization that incorporated a range of feeling states, and the therapist invited her to place the coloured sand on the various places in her body where she felt them. Stephanie really engaged with and enjoyed these activities and began journaling at home about her emotions – she even included a smaller version of the sensory gingerbread man in her journal. She shared these journal entries in her therapy sessions.

*Small world play*

Another major shift occurred at this stage: Stephanie began to give narratives to her creations in the sandtray. She would create miniature worlds, sometimes with a self-selected theme and sometimes with a theme suggested by the therapist. She would name the worlds and write a story to accompany each one. Personally relevant themes and stories continued to emerge, and Stephanie's ability to identify and name emotions and link emotional states to experiences developed further.

Throughout the therapeutic process, Stephanie did not speak to the therapist – she didn't need to. She did begin to speak to her friends at home, her teachers and her friends and peers in school. Aunts, uncles and cousins who had never heard her speak now recognized the sound of her voice. Stephanie no longer suffered from the emotional dysregulation that had caused her 'meltdowns' or feared going into a shop and not being able to order the sandwich she wanted. She now existed in a world where she could openly communicate with herself, others and the world around her.

## Maeve, age 20.2 years

Maeve was in her first year of university when she referred herself to creative psychotherapy. She reported that she was suffering from anxiety and that her symptoms had started a few weeks into her first semester in university. Each morning, when she arrived at university, she would begin to panic, her hands became sweaty, her heart would pound so much that it felt to her like it was going to 'burst', and she would hyperventilate. These symptoms had escalated so much that Maeve had begun skipping lectures and avoiding college friends. Maeve also noted that she was not sleeping well anymore and that she no longer felt hungry and was eating out of necessity rather than desire. When Maeve arrived for her first therapy session, she appeared highly anxious – she avoided eye contact, her hands were clammy, she was experiencing difficulty breathing and she repeatedly tapped her feet against the floor.

Maeve's presenting symptoms indicated a persistent fear state that was serious enough to prevent her from getting on with her everyday life. Trauma specialists describe how, in response to threatened survival, our primitive, reptilian brain (the brainstem and diencephalon) triggers the sympathetic nervous system into a fight/flight response, resulting in a hormonal rush of chemicals that prioritize the body's need to run away or fight back, shutting down the visceral digestive organs until the threat has passed and a release of cortisol signals a return to homeostasis (Rothschild, 2000; Perry, 2006; Levine and Kline, 2007; van der Kolk, 2014). In cases of extreme fear that has not been processed, or early developmental trauma, when the child experiences chronic threat, the body cannot recover, the nervous system is in a permanent state of fear arousal, and the body is flooded with cortisol, which, if constantly present, is corrosive to brain cells and results in hyperactivity of the fear system of the primitive brainstem (Panksepp and Biven, 2012), providing a fear state template for all feelings, thoughts and actions.

In accordance with the principles of the NMT (Perry, 2006), the therapist decided that she would initially need to focus her work on regulating Maeve's chronic anxiety state by providing a safe, trustworthy therapeutic relationship and introducing her to repetitive, rhythmic and sensory play-based activities.

Maeve engaged well with the sensory materials and, in particular, was drawn to the shells, sensory balls and fidgety toys. The therapist provided her with a stress ball and a fidgety toy on a key ring to take home. Maeve began carrying the stress ball in her college bag and keeping the key ring in an easily accessible pocket. She used them when she noticed her breathing changing or her heart beginning to race. Once she was shown what to do and had experienced the soothing, regulatory properties of the sensory play materials, she was able to use her tertiary brain thinking skills to act in order to soothe herself and regulate her anxiety symptoms before they overwhelmed her.

She was particularly drawn to the drumming activities and also moving to music. Initially, the therapist led these activities, creating co-regulation mirror games – she would direct and orchestrate the activity, and Maeve would follow. As the sessions progressed, Maeve began to engage freely in both the drumming and movement-based activities and would lead the sessions herself, integrating the therapist's sensitive response to her initiatives and becoming aware of her own innate pace, rhythm and flow.

During the middle stage of Maeve's therapy, the therapist introduced activities to promote and practise deep breathing. She used bubbles, balloons and guided imagery to encourage Maeve to focus on and gain control of her breathing and to help her to relax. Once again, Maeve integrated what she had learnt in therapy about regulating herself and she began using the deep-breathing techniques as she travelled to college and guided imagery to help herself to fall asleep at night.

During this stage of therapy Maeve began exploring the sandtray. She would play with dry sand, sometimes with eyes open and sometimes with closed eyes, without adding symbols. After eight therapy sessions, Maeve reported that she was no longer experiencing overwhelming panic and anxiety. Her sleeping had improved, and her appetite had returned. She felt she would be ready to finish after our twelve pre-contracted sessions. During her final four sessions, Maeve continued to engage in the drumming and movement activities and requested to finish each session with a creative visualization. She progressed to adding symbols and miniatures and creating stories in the sand. In her final session, she created 'Maeve's world' in the sandtray, a world containing a bottle of bubbles, a drum, some seashells and a sensory ball.

## Conclusion

The case studies show how an integrative, person-centred therapist with a thorough understanding of development, and sensitivity to the particular history and presenting issues of each client, can effectively incorporate sensory-based play into her practice.

## Key points

- Sensory play involves and integrates all the senses.
- Sensory integration is fundamental to self-regulation and healthy brain development.
- Therapeutic interventions that provide a full spectrum of sensory play enable clients to have access to experiences that are helpful in calming or stimulating the nervous system.
- Sensory play regulates brainstem and midbrain reactivity.

## References

Ayres, J.A. (2005). *Sensory Integration and the Child: Understanding hidden sensory challenges* (25th Anniversary edn). Los Angeles, CA: Western Psychological Services.

Beckerleg, T. (2009). *Fun with Messy Play: Ideas and activities for children with special needs*. London: Jessica Kingsley.

Bemis, K. (2014). Stress management. In C.E. Schaefer and A.A. Drewes (eds) *The Therapeutic Powers of Play: 20 core agents of change* (2nd edn; pp. 143–52). Hoboken, NJ: Wiley.

Booth, P.B., and Jernberg, A.M. (2010). *Theraplay: Helping parents and children build better relationships through attachment-based play* (3rd edn). San Francisco, CA: John Wiley.

Bruce, T. (2011). *Learning Through Play for Babies, Toddlers and Young Children* (2nd edn). London: Hodder Education.

Cozolino, L. (2010). *The Neuroscience of Psychotherapy: Healing the social brain*. New York: W.W. Norton.

Fearn, M. (2014). Working therapeutically with groups in the outdoors: A natural space for healing. In E. Prendiville and J. Howard (eds) *Play Therapy Today: Contemporary practice for individuals, groups and carers* (pp. 7–28). London: Routledge.

Frank, R. (2001). *Body of Awareness: A somatic and developmental approach to psychotherapy*. Cambridge, MA: Gestalt Press.

Gascoyne, S. (2012). *Treasure Baskets and Beyond: Realizing the potential of sensory-rich play*. Maidenheaad, UK: Open University Press.

Gaskill, R. (2014). Empathy. In C.E. Schaefer and A.A. Drewes (eds) *The Therapeutic Powers of Play: 20 core agents of change* (2nd edn; pp. 195–207). Hoboken, NJ: Wiley.

Gerhardt, S. (2004). *Why Love Matters: How affection shapes a baby's brain*. New York: Brunner-Routledge.

Gil, E. (2013). Integrating a neurosequential approach in the treatment of traumatized children, Part II. Interview with C.F. Sori and S. Schnur. *The Family Journal: Counselling & Therapy for Couples & Families*. DOI: 10.1177/1066480713514945.

Godwin Emmons, P., and McKendry Anderson, L. (2005). *Understanding Sensory Dysfunction: Learning, development and sensory dysfunction in autism spectrum disorders, ADHD, learning disabilities and bipolar disorder*. London: Jessica Kingsley.

Goldschmied, E., and Jackson, S. (1994). *People Under Three: Young children in daycare*. London: Routledge.

Huttenlocher, P.R. (2002). *Neural Plasticity: The effects of environment on the development of the cerebral cortex*. Cambridge, MA: Harvard University Press.

Jennings, S. (1999). *Introduction to Developmental Playtherapy*. London: Jessica Kingsley.

Jennings, S. (2011). *Healthy Attachments and Neuro-Dramatic Play*. London: Jessica Kingsley.

Jennings, S. (2014). Applying an Embodiment–Projection–Role framework in groupwork with children. In E. Prendiville and J. Howard (eds) *Play Therapy Today: Contemporary practice for individuals, groups and carers* (pp. 81–96). London: Routledge.

Levine, P.A. and Kline, M. (2007). *Trauma Through a Child's Eyes. Awakening the ordinary miracle of healing*. Berkeley, CA: North Atlantic Books.

McCune-Nicolich, L. (1977). Beyond sensorimotor intelligence: Assessment of symbolic maturity through analysis of pretend play. *Merrill-Palmer Quarterly*, 23, 89–99.

Munns, E. (2014). Group Theraplay. In E. Prendiville and J. Howard (eds) *Play Therapy Today: Contemporary practice for individuals, groups and carers* (pp. 163–78). London: Routledge.
Panksepp, J., and Biven, L. (2012). *The Archaeology of Mind: Neuroevolutionary origins of human emotions.* New York: W.W. Norton.
Perry, B.D. (2006). Applying principles of neurodevelopment to clinical work with maltreated and traumatized children. In N. Webb (ed.) *Working with Traumatized Youth in Child Welfare* (pp. 27–52). New York: Guilford Press.
Perry, B.D., Hogan, L., and Marlin, S.J. (2000). Curiosity, pleasure and play: A neuro-developmental perspective. *Haaeyc Advocate,* 9–12.
Piaget, J. (1954). *The Construction of Reality in the Child.* New York: Basic Books.
Piaget, J. (1964). Development and learning. Part 1: Cognitive development in children. *Journal of Research in Science Teaching,* 2(Sept), 176–86.
Porges, S.W. (2011). In conversation with Serge Prengel (transcription). Somatic Perspectives on Psychotherapy Series. Available at: www.SomaticPerspectives.com (accessed 30 May 2016).
Prendiville, E. (2014a). The therapeutic touchstone. In E. Prendiville and J. Howard (eds) *Play Therapy Today: Contemporary practice for individuals, groups and carers* (pp. 7–28). London: Routledge.
Prendiville, E. (2014b). Abreaction. In C.E. Schaefer and A.A. Drewes (eds) *The Therapeutic Powers of Play: 20 core agents of change* (2nd edn; pp. 83–103). Hoboken, NJ: Wiley.
Prendiville, S. (2014). Accelerated psychological development. In C.E. Schaefer and A.A. Drewes (eds) *The Therapeutic Powers of Play: 20 core agents of change* (2nd edn; pp. 255–68). Hoboken, NJ: Wiley.
Pulaski, M.A. (1976). Play symbolism in cognitive development. In C.E. Schaefer (ed.) *Therapeutic Use of Child's Play* (pp. 27–41). New York: Jason Aronson.
Rothschild, B. (2000). *The Body Remembers: The Psychophysiology of Trauma and Trauma Treatment.* New York: W.W. Norton.
Schore, A.N. (2005). Attachment, affect and the developing right brain: Linking developmental neuroscience to pediatrics. *Pediatric Review, 26,* 204–17.
Schore, J., and Schore, A. (2008). Modern attachment theory: The central role of affect regulation in development and treatment. *Clinical Social Work Journal, 36,* 9–20.
Stagnitti, K. (1998). *Learn to Play: A practical program to develop a child's imaginative play skills.* Melbourne, VIC: Co-ordinates.
Stagnitti, K. (2009). Play intervention – The learn to play program. In K. Stagnitti and R. Cooper (eds) *Play as Therapy* (pp. 178–86). London: Jessica Kingsley.
Stern, D.N. (1985). *The Interpersonal World of the Infant: A view from psychoanalysis and developmental psychology.* New York: Basic Books.
Tassoni, P., and Hucker, K. (2005). *Planning Play and the Early Years.* Oxford, UK: Heinemann.
van der Kolk, B. (2014). *The Body Keeps the Score: Brain, mind and body in the healing of trauma.* New York: Penguin.
West, C. (2011). The Just Right State Programme. Service evaluation – Executive summary (PDF). Available at: www.sensoryattachmentintervention.com/Documents/Just%20Right%20State%20Programme%20Executive%20Summary.pdf (accessed 2 December 2015).

Williamson, G.G., and Anzalone, M. (1997). Sensory integration: A key component of the evaluation and treatment of young children with severe difficulties in relating and communicating. *Zero to Three, 17*(5), 29–36.

# Part III

# Working with the limbic and cortical systems

The infant experiences the world and relationships through their senses. In Part II, the role of sensory interventions, music and rhythm, and movement and touch has been examined relative to the earliest developing areas of the brain, the brainstem and midbrain. As interventions, they do not rely on verbal language or written symbols. Rather, they use the senses to calm the stress response, provide a felt sense of safety and provide reparative experiences of nurturance and empathic attunement. Sensory play is fundamental to self-regulation, providing both stimulation and calming, and regulates midbrain reactivity. As the case scenarios illustrated, using sensory interventions in play does not limit the positive effects to the lower brain regions, but provides the base and is flexible to allow therapy to progress to the next neurodevelopmental level. In Part III, work with the limbic and cortical areas will be explored – promoting emotional growth, developing fluidity between body and mind and promoting self-expression, self-awareness and insight.

Chapter 8

# Art in psychotherapy
The healing power of images

*Claire Colreavy Donnelly*

The chapter describes art in psychotherapy and art psychotherapy and contextualizes these approaches within relevant theoretical models of neurobiology. It locates the use of art within a neurosequential framework and illustrates approaches to working with adults, adolescents and children who have experienced emotional distress, trauma or loss. Working with the unconscious, limbic resonance and affect regulation are key overlapping themes that are explored by using case material to highlight how effective art psychotherapy is as an intervention that enables client recovery by working with limbic and cortical systems of the brain. It demonstrates how the practice facilitates therapeutic attunement, affect expression and affect regulation. It is proposed that art in psychotherapy is an effective tool that, by engaging clients in creative activities, builds inner resources, promotes brain plasticity and offers strategies for ongoing self-care.

Art helps clients externalize their internal realities. Through the use of art in creative psychotherapies, the reflexive loop that exists between how we perceive life (our internal dialogues) and the impact this has on our external reality can be worked with explicitly through clients being helped to creatively project their thoughts and feelings on to a map of themselves and their world. Once externalized, this imagery offers more possibility for therapist attunement and helps clients test reality, gaining objectivity, insight and power over the projected material. It is this unique process of creative projection and subsequent introjection that creates the possibility of therapeutic change. Neurobiological concepts overlap with key principles of art psychotherapy, namely working with the unconscious, limbic resonance and affect regulation.

Wood (1998) explains that it is more appropriate to define art psychotherapy as the approach used within the profession of art therapy: 'It is what Art Therapists do'. The practice is informed by psychoanalysis, psychotherapy, developmental psychology and, more recently, neuroscience. Art psychotherapy is a form of psychotherapy where a triangular relationship exists between therapist, client and artwork or image. Images can be created through the use of traditional art materials, but also through the use of figurines, found objects, mixed media or the use of the client's own body in the therapeutic space. As an art psychotherapist, I expand the therapeutic frame to include everything that may take place within the session, as this can also be read as an image symbolically and offer material to help develop therapeutic attunement. Alongside the therapeutic alliance, there is the client's expression of their own creativity, which is invested with personal meaning and symbolism. Art psychotherapy works with unconscious processes by encouraging clients to create images while engaged in a state of reverie or creative free association. What is produced as a third point of contact has a strong relational component, meaningfully engaging the client interpersonally and intrapersonally through mind–body connections, in order to create a map of their experience.

'In the art therapist's presence, the art work is an expression of how the self organizes internally as well as in relationship with others. It is a visual reiteration of the interplay between the person and their environment' (Hass-Cohen, 2008: 21).

In offering access to this material, art offers clients a way to project their inner experience, helping them to feel understood and accepted through therapeutic attunement, limbic resonance and containment. Therapists also provide experiences for clients to explore and meet themselves in new ways by engaging with their artwork. This engagement has the potential to help them gain flexibility in terms of finding new attachment narratives and in offering them live situations where they can rehearse different ways of responding to psychic material. The experimentation and rehearsal have the power to impact on brain plasticity and to support self-regulation by providing new ways to help clients cope with overwhelming feelings and experience therapeutic change.

## The unconscious

Jung (1916) believed imagery to be the language of the unconscious and described his reasons for inviting his patients to paint: 'the aim of this method of expression is to make unconscious contents accessible and so bring them closer to the patient's understanding' (quoted in Schaverien, 1992: 81). Freud explained that, 'thinking in pictures . . . stands nearer to unconscious processes than does thinking in words' (1923: 21). Mental processes differ in quality, some being conscious, others unconscious. Freud described how unconscious processes, those that the subject is not aware of, can directly influence emotional and behavioural affect and interpersonal relationships. He created useful psychoanalytic concepts that help us understand unconscious processes and human psychological functioning. Within psychoanalysis, transference is the process by which a patient unconsciously transfers feelings and ideas from a significant relationship on to the therapist. In art psychotherapy, the client can also transfer significant feelings and ideas on to their artwork, which can be worked with in order to gain self-awareness. Bowlby's attachment theory (1969), showing how the primary relationship experienced by the child with their caregiver is formative and creates an attachment pattern that can become an implicit template for future relationships, connects with Freud's concept of transference. It can be argued that the field of neuroscience has incorporated both of these concepts by speaking of 'patterns in the mind that have developed as a result of early and subsequent experience ... which are stored in implicit memory' (Wilkinson, 2010: 58). These brain patterns or internal working models can serve as markers for future interpersonal relationships and are readily made visible within artwork. When implicit patterns become explicit through the creation of pictorial records, these records or artworks can provide insight and an opportunity for the client/artist to experiment and alter or adapt their responses to them.

Art psychotherapy places a greater emphasis on nonverbal, non-linguistic areas of therapeutic work and, through the use of image, engages aspects of implicit memory. The unconscious, memory and image are related. In the first 3 years of life, the right-brain hemisphere develops before left functions come online. Autobiographical, implicit memories, encoded as images, are stored in the unconscious mind before conscious, explicit memory begins to evolve with the development of language expression and comprehension at 18 months:

> Implicit memory does not require conscious awareness. It directs actions, reactions and body responses with little or no conscious effort, involving multiple brain structures. Implicit memories refer to somatic/bodily, perceptual experiences, which include memories of how things looked or smelled as well as our emotions and moods at the time.
> (Vance and Wahlin, 2008: 162)

With its focus on the use of materials that facilitate somatosensory engagement, art in psychotherapy provides a powerful route into the unconscious. When clients access unconscious material by the safe expression of latent imagery, their self-awareness and personal insight can deepen. Therapists need to be alert to any signs that a client is becoming triggered by the use of materials that are particularly evocative to them. Therapeutic safety and containment through the use of established boundaries and a trusting therapeutic alliance should always be a prerequisite for inviting clients to engage with emotionally charged material. Therapeutic reassurance for the client and consolidation of state regulation can create a secure enough base from which clients may find it possible to self-regulate and process the work further by thinking about it.

Creative expression is more engaged with right-brain functioning and can be worked with in both a bottom–up – unconscious led – and top–down – conscious led – approach. For example working in a somatosensory way, we can encourage a client to connect with and express feelings about their family through the selection and use of certain materials because of these materials' innate qualities, that is, softness or sharpness. This engages a more unconscious, implicit-memory, bottom–up approach. On the other hand, offering a clear directive for a client to make an image of their family from thinking about their role within it employs a top–down, more conscious approach. In the former, we are helping the client access emotional material by using their senses, through midbrain on to limbic and then to cortical levels. 'Personal symbolic art expression most likely allows sensory routes to speak directly to the limbic brain' (Clyde Findlay, 2008: 214). When emotions are accessed and expressed in this way, they can then become available for sorting and processing by being brought into the thinking, cortical level. In the case of the latter example, we initially engage the client's thinking processes, which in turn become illustrations or descriptions. This more conscious approach creates representations that fall into the category of diagrammatic images, classified by the analytic art psychotherapist Schaverien as 'usually an approximation of a preconceived mental image' and 'an illustration or a description of a feeling but it is not an embodiment' (Schaverien, 1992: 86). These images act as maps to communicate information, but they do not hold the power of embodied images. Embodied images tend to engage the client's unconscious in a more holistic way, employing a fuller mind–body connection that can help them transform and shift psychic blocks: 'The embodied picture transcends what is consciously known' (Schaverien, 1992: 87). When this kind of artwork is subsequently engaged with by being thought about, spoken about and processed in a multidirectional way – that is, bottom–up and bilaterally, from left- to right-brain systems – more integration can take place. The use of symbolism and metaphor helps us develop integration by connecting left- and right-brain systems: 'The symbolic image is generated by the dual processes of the mind. It depends upon dynamic synergism between left and right hemisphere. It is the optimal balancing of imagery, emotion and thought which facilitates the creative process' (Cox and Theilgaard, 1997: 137).

## Limbic resonance and intersubjectivity

The limbic system is a conceptual, rather than anatomical, designation used to group central brain structures that regulate, evaluate and integrate emotion into motivational states, survival responses and memories (Schore, 2012). Perception and emotional learning in the area of attunement arise out of our earliest relationships. Emotional resonance and attunement by the primary caregiver offer experiences for co-regulation and meaning-making. This intersubjective experience becomes the blueprint for interpersonal relationships and is termed the internal working model. Schore's work in the field of infant mental health and Stern's work on intersubjectivity (1985) place importance on the right-brain-to-right-brain communication within the mother–infant relationship and the effect of this on brain development. Because, as Bowlby (1988) states, the therapeutic relationship can reactivate patients' unconscious expectations about responsiveness and availability of others, therapists need to create a safe, containing environment and a strong therapeutic alliance by engaging in right-brain-to-right-brain sensitivity to their clients. In simple terms, Schore describes the left-brain system as having a thinking function, with the right brain related to emotional processing. He talks about the left and right hemispheres of the brain as two cortical–subcortical systems with unique structure and functions. He makes the distinction between how emotion is processed within the brain, describing the left as the linguistic brain dealing with secondary-process functioning, working with conscious, rational thought and explicit memory: what he terms Freud's Ego. The right brain he terms the social–emotional brain, dealing with primary-process functioning, working with the unconscious, implicit memory and self-systems: Freud's Id (Schore, 2012).

Schore helps us locate our practice by identifying which aspects of brain functioning we seek to work with and how we might achieve our clinical goals of therapeutic attunement and limbic resonance. Like Bowlby's theories of attachment (1969) and Bion's work on therapeutic containment (1962), Schore discusses the importance of the role of the primary caregiver in helping develop and shape the infant's core sense of self. He notes the paradigm shift in therapy from 'working with the explicit, analytical, conscious, verbal, rational left hemisphere' to that of 'the implicit, integrative, unconscious, nonverbal, bodily based emotional right hemisphere' (Schore, 2012: 7). He cautions against focusing exclusively on verbal exchanges while neglecting nonverbal behaviour in the therapeutic process. When therapists work with creative, mind–body, integrative, implicit approaches, we work with right-brain-to-right-brain communication. In this, we can achieve limbic resonance with a client, which helps them feel understood and contained. This attunement is a prerequisite for helping clients gain a sense of safety from which they can move on to express difficult feelings and develop some sense of control or mastery over them.

## Affect regulation

Diener *et al.*'s clinical research (2007) shows that therapists' affect facilitation is a powerful predictor of treatment success. When the therapist encourages the client to create images, these images become external representations of the client's internal realities. This facilitates affect expression through engaging with the client's limbic system. It can then offer subsequent affect regulation by helping the client pass this raw emotion, once expressed and objectified, into a kind of sorting, naming and meaning-making process within the cortical system. Once affect has been expressed, the client can be helped to explore personal meanings within their work by engaging bilateral systems through the use of symbolism and metaphor. Working with metaphor can have a containing and integrative effect on clients and offer opportunities for change. Pally (2000), quoted in Wilkinson (2010), says, 'Such metaphors stimulate brain activity in a more thorough way; such processing, utilizing as it does brain plasticity, brings with it more possibility of change than any other form of human communication' (p. 113).

When safety and a sense of trust are established, the client is encouraged to work, in the spirit of play and experimentation, with the plasticity of the art or self object. This can become a powerful process that highlights the client's sense of ownership, choice and mastery over their work and therefore, by analogy, over the difficulties they face in life. Becoming an agent of change is evidenced both physiologically and psychologically in the work by a client who engages in this personal feedback loop. A reflexive process takes place when clients practise externalizing psychic material through projective work, when they exert choice over the creative alterations they wish to make to this, and when they re-introject this new material through their senses. This process has the effect of changing inner dialogues by changing external reality. Previous mental and emotional associations can be re-routed, effecting brain plasticity by helping the client form new sensory pathways and symbolic links. Bilateral brain connections are formed through the use of metaphor when clients bridge emotional affect with what makes sense for them in a different way.

In understanding the link between how we perceive and receive images, Achterberg (1985) summarizes general research findings on imagery and physiology:

> Images relate to physiological states; images may either precede or follow physiological changes, indicating both a causal or reactive role; images may be induced by conscious, deliberate behaviours, as well as by subconscious acts (electrical stimulation of the brain, reverie, dreaming etc.); images can be considered as the hypothetical bridge between conscious processing of information and physiological change; images can exhibit influence over the voluntary (peripheral) nervous system, as well as the involuntary (autonomic) nervous system.
>
> (p. 115)

Harnessing the powerful effect that images have on our physiological states within art psychotherapy and art in psychotherapy can be a very effective treatment approach (see Colreavy Donnelly, 2010).

## Neurosequential considerations

In Perry's model (2006: 41), the limbic and cortical systems are associated with the development and regulation of emotional states that are connected with play and creative activities involving mark-making, symbolism, pretence and social interaction. Although, within art psychotherapy, the main focus may be on working with these higher brain systems, the practice can inhabit all four levels of Perry's schema, working initially with brainstem systems to establish state regulation by helping the client feel safe within therapy through therapeutic containment and the establishment of boundaries. This relates to Bannister's first R of reassurance (described in Chapter 2), provided by the use of the therapist's body language, tone of voice, warmth and prosodic communication. If successful, this in turn provides an experience of a secure enough base, which helps the client navigate through difficult and sometimes overwhelming psychic material. Midbrain systems can be employed in helping clients incorporate somatosensory integration by experimenting with art materials in a self-soothing and rhythmical way. This therapeutic assistance can help a client to regulate their physiology if they are experiencing overwhelming symptoms of dysregulation. It is important for the therapist to attune to the client and discern which level they are functioning at in order to intervene or direct the therapy effectively.

As the first two areas of brain functioning are worked with and a sense of relational stability, trust and safety ensues, the introduction of strategies aimed at engaging the limbic system can aid emotional regulation. Encouraging clients to connect with, embody and project confusing feelings and thoughts promotes catharsis and helps develop insight. Once difficulties have been objectified and expressed, their scale can be put into perspective through the client's use of movement and position in relation to their artwork. They can be encouraged to take up different spectator positions while they speak to a chosen aspect of the work. This process of being able to simultaneously inhabit and connect with difficult psychic material expressed through artwork, while also speaking to it from within different internal roles, can help clients exert an element of control that aids emotional regulation and healing.

Experiences of emotional distress, trauma or loss may contribute to affect dysregulation and distorted thinking and can create a discontinuity of being (Winnicott, 1958), which is destabilizing. These internal experiences of chaos, fragmentation or emptiness affect identity, relationships and how we respond to life. Within a safe therapeutic relationship, when internal experience is creatively expressed in concrete terms and witnessed by an attuned therapist, the client can experience a sense of integration and containment. Simple acts, such as when the therapist directs the client to make a physical container to house their work and provides safe storage for this, can help the client feel held and secure.

## Adult client: Mary

When clients come to therapy having experienced trauma, offering them verbal psychotherapy alone can become a re-traumatizing experience. Because trauma is stored in the body and has a physiological basis, when they try to communicate their experience, clients' neocortical brain functions can become flooded with affect, making it impossible for them to think clearly, gain insight or self-regulate.

Mary, a middle-aged widow with adult children, worked in the care system. She experienced a traumatic motor accident while at work. She was seated in the back of an ambulance alone, having escorted a patient to hospital, when the ambulance crashed. Mary was violently thrown as the vehicle careered forwards and backwards until it came to a stop. She experienced feelings of panic and thoughts of death. She initially appeared to cope well, but later described 'a kind of beside myself feeling'. It was only after she drove herself home and was coming to her doorstep that she collapsed and felt the full force of symptoms of shock. Since then, her sleep and food intake had been severely disrupted. She had flashbacks of the incident, with the accompanying symptoms of fear and panic, sometimes triggered by the sound of sirens or seeing an ambulance, but often when preparing for bed at night. The regular occurence of waking in fear, with cold sweats, caused her further fragility by blocking any attempt at state regulation by finding nourishment through sleep. Mary appeared in a state of hypervigilance, unable to access any feelings of internal safety.

> If a deeply traumatised person is prompted only to speak and think about the events that created his distress, without enlisting help from the imaginal, emotional, sensory, and somatic capabilities of his right brain, his symptoms can actually get worse instead of better [. . .] methods are needed that can blessedly sidestep the booby-trapped language centres in the brain by making clever use of imaginal, multisensory, motor, and emotional pathways – pathways that are in a heightened state of receptivity, due to the very same biochemical hit that disabled the capacity for words in the first place . . . imagery uses what is most accessible in the traumatised brain to help with the healing.
>
> (Naparstek, 2006: XVIII)

I established a therapeutic relationship with Mary by encouraging her to relate her experience while I offered her soothing sensory activity. I suggested she let dry sand fall through her fingers as she retold her experience. For some clients this could be too irritating, as their senses become hypersensitive, but for Mary this seemed to have a distracting effect that diluted the feelings of overwhelm that she had experienced previously when being asked to report the accident. I believe this somatosensory activity helped re-route some of the physiological memories captured in her body from the incident.

In subsequent sessions, I asked Mary to create an image through small world objects and materials that created a feeling of safety inside. With encouragement, she chose a small figure of a female child and created a nest, surrounding her with soft feathers (see Figure 8.1). I asked her to talk to the figure in a reassuring way, helping her to feel safe. This became an emotionally laden experience that was very touching. In creative therapies, we talk about the 'as if' moments, which bring profound meaning and healing by helping the client inhabit two places at once. Through this form of aesthetic distancing, Mary was identifying with both the vulnerability and brokeness of the child and the containing empathic presence of a strong internal adult. She spoke in soft, caring tones and witnessed hearing herself saying aloud what she most needed to hear inside when she felt the terror of her experience being reactivated. I encouraged her to practise this way of speaking aloud and of becoming conscious of how it made her breathe more deeply and calmly. I asked her permission to take a photograph of her image for her to keep as a concrete record: a kind of 'image medication' that she could look at in order to be reminded of her current sensations and sense of containment. When Mary did this in my presence, I believe something shifted in her because I could vouch for the healthy aspect of herself that was capable of taking charge. Mary reported using this image regularly, keeping it by her pillow for when she might awake at night in panic.

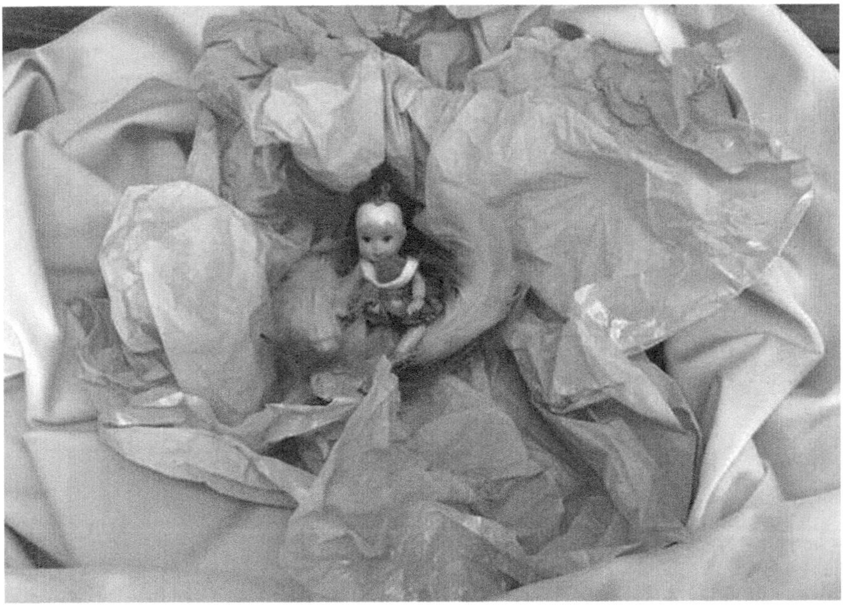

*Figure 8.1* Mary: Safe space

In subsequent sessions, once she had accessed and practised this strategy for self-care, I asked her to explore alternative associations or memories that she might have of ambulances. In this way, I was moving up from working with her limbic system to engaging her on a cortical level by harnessing her conscious memories. She recalled a beautiful memory of having escorted an elderly man, in an ambulance, to meet his wife at a nursing home in which they were both now going to reside. I asked her to visualize this and become conscious of all the sensory details around this experience. Her body language changed, and she became visibly relaxed and calm. She smiled and by now knew that this was what she needed to, if not replace, at least connect with as a simultaneous association, to help balance the previous traumatic memory and experience. Mary's therapy lasted eight sessions. At the follow-up on her progress after 2 years, she gave the following feedback: 'It was a life saver, something so simple and it worked. I could have been going to doctors being put on medication, but I didn't want that. I still have the postcard. It helped a lot'.

## Adolescent client: Alice

Alice came to art psychotherapy as part of a discharge programme from an adolescent inpatient unit. Although her mental health had stabilized, and she was no longer actively suicidal, she was, however, still deliberately self-harming. Alice regularly engaged in cutting herself on her thighs, chest and arms. Having built up a therapeutic alliance with her, I worked explicitly with Alice around this behaviour by encouraging her to explore creative alternatives. I invited her to use clay and try to connect safely, through the use of aesthetic distance, with feelings she associated with her self-harm. I asked her to 'act out' on the clay the way she would with her own body. Alice initially created a curious shape that to me looked like a large spoon. She then began adding fingers to the form, which made it look more like an arm (see Figure 8.2), and later slashed the arm repeatedly with a sharp clay tool. Although engaged intensely with this work, she did not appear to

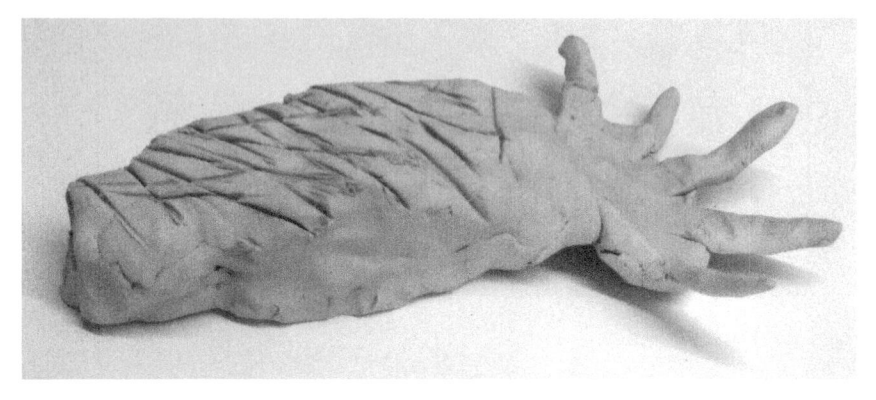

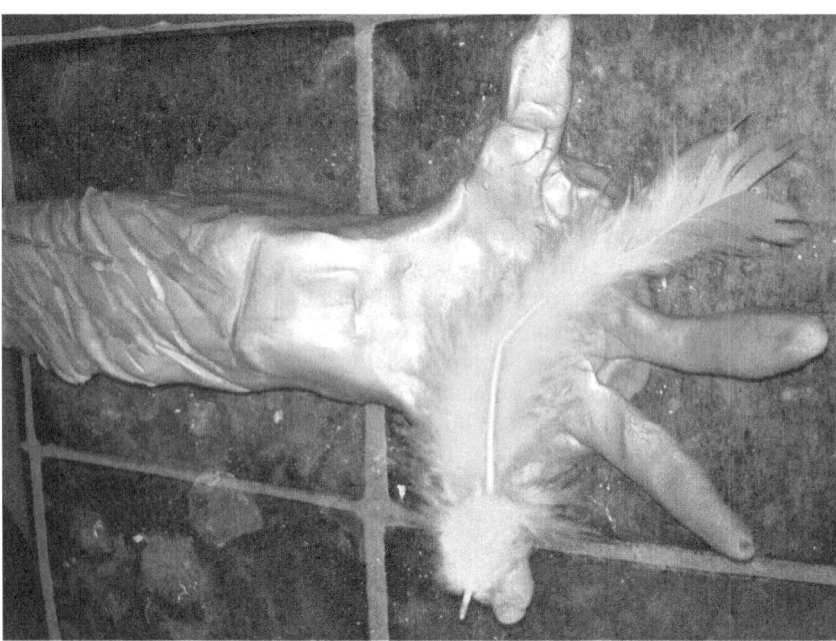

*Figure 8.2* Alice: Sore arm

become overwhelmed but seemed to achieve some kind of catharsis through the activity by ridding herself of something burdensome. She appeared relieved and tired after this experience.

I encouraged Alice to share her work and her experience of engaging in this activity. She explained that somehow, through playing with and feeling the clay, she had remembered incidents where her parent had punished her for bad behaviour by hitting her with a wooden spoon. She had followed this memory by recreating an external form in the shape of a wooden spoon. She then turned this shape into an image of her arm and later continued expressing this internal association by doing what felt familiar to her: she slashed her arm. Once she had projected out this narrative, it seemed she was capable of wondering about this chain of events. She appeared able to move her experience up into a thinking place and made the connections between her feelings of being bad and shameful and needing to be punished. I asked her whether she wanted to continue making and feeling these associations or whether she would like to ask the arm what it needed. She appeared capable of finding empathy with her sculpture while simultaneously being able to stay separate enough in order to engage in a healthy dialogue with this aspect of herself. She answered that the sore arm needed care. I asked her how she might be able to offer this, and very spontaneously she chose a yellow feather and started to rythmically stroke it. I asked her what kind of sensory and emotional feedback she felt from this experience, and she said, 'it feels good' and became more relaxed and calm. I encouraged Alice to try to continue to be open to this new feedback and to practise giving the sore arm what it needed.

Alice experimented with the plasticity of her artwork but also with the plasticity of her physical and emotional responses to the memories and associations that the artwork elicited from her. I believe that with this work, alongside her usual psychological associations, she began to change some of the somatosensory and neuronal pathways previously laid down, by creating a new feedback loop between her senses, her memories, her feelings and her new experiences. The measurement of this, as with Mary, was evidenced in the positive physiological changes that were witnessed by the therapist in Alice at the time and by subsequent reports that while in therapy she had disengaged from self-harm.

## Child clients: David and Leonie

David was 8 years old and in foster care at the time of therapy. He had a difficult history, having experienced three different placements. David presented as highly dysregulated, finding it difficult to settle in school and in the new placement. He would sometimes show a lot of compliance, as if trying desperately to be 'a good boy' in order to be cared for, but then a build-up of internal anxiety and tension would burst out and cause disruption, shame and guilt. David was very defensive. With a therapeutic alliance having been tentatively built, it seemed very important for him to experience a caring adult witnessing and understanding his reality. One of the first images he created was the image in Figure 8.3.

152  Claire Colreavy Donnelly

David described this in an offhand way as 'just someone who feels crazy'. In this image, I think David really helps us understand what it might feel like to have a sensory processing disorder that can feel overwhelming. The figure, he explained, 'has lots of ears, eyes, noses, mouths and feels too much'. This image helped me attune to David's experience and also, I believe, not only helped him feel understood by me but created a visual map of his experience through which

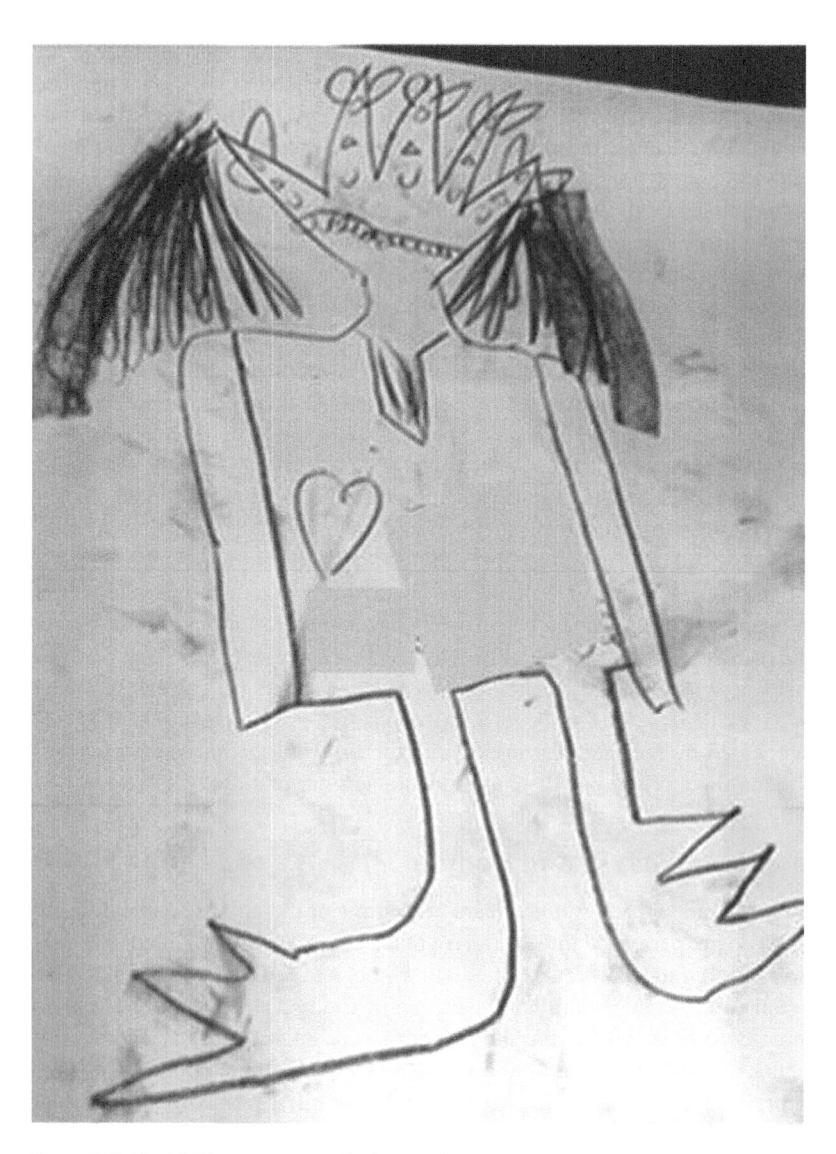

*Figure 8.3* David: 'Someone who feels crazy'

he could begin to find insight into himself. I responded in an equally offhand way, speaking out to the space as opposed to him directly, saying, 'it was no wonder if this person used some armour to get by – feeling this way must be very difficult to control'. He agreed in a distracted way, and I encouraged him to see what might help this figure feel calm. He broke away and began playing with dry sand. This appeared to have a soothing effect on David, and I reflected how resourceful he could be in finding his own way of 'calming the crazy'. This experience helped create a shared language between us and also helped David to articulate how he might be feeling. Whether he might feel like he needed to be in his armoured place or whether he might be open to self-soothing could be explored with him. In future sessions with David, if he felt overwhelmed, I would remind him of this technique.

Leonie, a 10-year-old girl, had difficulties coming to terms with her parents' separation. At one point, she appeared very agitated, and so I asked her if she would like to do something soothing. She agreed, and I invited her to experiment with a favourite colour of paint and see if she could massage the paper with it. She became curious, and I showed her this technique, demonstrating using my hands to spread paint in circular motions. She did this and appeared to find some relief in the activity (see Figure 8.4). The interesting thing about this image, on reflection, is its sense of duality in terms of how it shows the marks of both hands moving together, engaging both sides of the body and integrating them as one

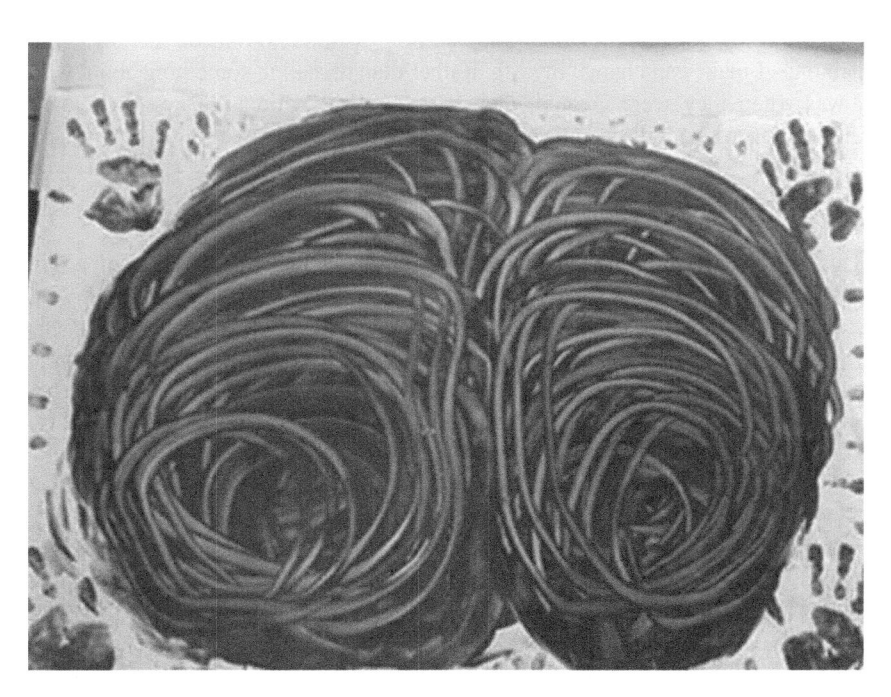

*Figure 8.4* Leonie: Self-soothing

movement/image. It also looks like the two brain hemsipheres. For Leonie, as with David, this activity helped her focus on her own self-soothing capacity and inner resourcefulness.

## Conclusion

This chapter explored the use of art psychotherapy and art in psychotherapy as a neurodevelopmentally appropriate intervention for adults, adolescents and children suffering from emotional distress, loss or trauma. It describes working with a client's limbic and cortical system to address the inner layers of damage. In helping clients connect with their emotional brokenness while also engaging their healthy selves, we help them create new attachment narratives to help replace old patterns. The case material presented illustrated how metaphorical images have the power to help clients gain insight into, and self-awareness of, their own process. Inviting clients to engage in simple self-soothing activities on a somatosensory level can help change their physiology and help regulate affect. The images appeared to simultaneously express aspects of client disregulation in terms of childhood fragility while also providing opportunities for clients' subsequent healing through their creative access to feelings of compassion, protection and agency. Art psychotherapy affords therapists opportunities to attune to clients and to gain limbic resonance with them.

In art psychotherapy, clients become creators of their own healing imagery, creating resources that they may draw on both within and outside therapy. 'The paintings I make can change my life. Rather than revealing something about who I was when they were created, the images will sometimes make a statement influencing who I will become' (McNiff, 1992: 64).

## Key points

This chapter has highlighted many benefits associated with the use of art in psychotherapy:

- It affords therapists opportunities to attune to clients and to gain limbic resonance with them.
- It is a means of self-expression, making visible the client's story or identity.
- It facilitates self-awareness and insight, making sense of experiences.
- It provides opportunities for clients to experiment safely – a way to practise seeing, thinking or feeling differently through new associations.
- It supports the development of new neural pathways and impacts positively on brain development.
- Is is an aid to emotional growth and development, helping clients articulate and name a range of emotions.
- As a method of connecting mind and body fluidly, it enhances well-being and supports integration.

- It supports emotional waste management, facilitating a form of catharsis where the client ventilates burdensome feelings and affect.
- It builds empowerment by allowing the client to exert control and gain mastery over artwork and, by analogy, personal difficulties.
- Through the rhythmic use of materials with calming properties, it allows for somatosensory self-soothing.
- By creating images that hold self-soothing properties in a symbolic way, it enhances the client's capacity for self-regulation (e.g. image medication).

## References

Achterberg, J. (1985). *Imagery in Healing, Shamanism and Modern Medicine.* Boston, MA: Shambhala.
Bion, W. (1962). *Learning from Experience.* London: Karnac.
Bowlby, J. (1969). *Attachment and Loss.* London: Hogarth Press.
Bowlby, J. (1988). *A Secure Base.* London: Routledge.
Clyde Findlay, J. (2008). Immunity at risk and art therapy. In N. Hass-Cohen and R. Carr (eds) *Art Therapy and Clinical Neuroscience* (pp. 207–22). London: Jessica Kingsley.
Colreavy Donnelly, C. (2010). The importance of image in the creative arts therapies. *Inside Out* (IAHIP), *61*(Summer).
Cox, M., and Theilgaard, A. (1997). *Mutative Metaphors in Psychotherapy: The Aeolian mode.* London: Jessica Kingsley.
Diener, M.J., Hilsenroth, M.J., and Weinberger, J. (2007). Therapist affect focus and patient outcomes in psychodynamic psychotherapy: A meta-analysis. *American Journal of Psychiatry*, *164*, 936–41.
Freud, S. (1923). *The Ego and the Id* (standard edn, vol. 19). London: Hogarth Press and Institute of Psychoanalysis.
Hass-Cohen, N. (2008). Partnering of art therapy and clinical neuroscience. In N. Hass-Cohen and R. Carr (eds) *Art Therapy and Clinical Neuroscience* (pp. 21–42). London: Jessica Kingsley.
Jung, C. (1916). *The Psychology of the Unconscious.* Mineola, NY: Dover.
McNiff, S. (1992). *Art as Medicine: Creating a therapy of the imagination.* Boston, MA: Shambhala.
Naparstek, B. (2006). *Invisible Heroes: Survivors of trauma and how they heal.* London: Piatkus.
Pally, R. (2000). *The Mind–Brain Relationship.* New York: Karnac.
Perry, B.D. (2006). The neurosequential model of therapeutics: Applying principles of neuroscience to clinical work with traumatized and maltreated children. In N.B. Webb (ed.) *Working with Traumatized Youth in Child Welfare* (pp. 27–52). New York: Guilford Press.
Schaverien, J. (1992). *The Revealing Image: Analytical art psychotherapy in theory and practice.* London: Jessica Kingsley.
Schore, A. (2012). *The Science of the Art of Psychotherapy.* New York: Norton.
Stern, D.N. (1985). *The Interpersonal World of the Infant: A view from psychoanalysis and Developmental Psychology.* New York: Basic Books.

Vance, R., and Wahlin, K. (2008). Memory and art. In N. Hass-Cohen and R. Carr (eds) *Art Therapy and Clinical Neuroscience* (pp. 159–73). London: Jessica Kingsley.

Wilkinson, M. (2010). *Changing Minds in Therapy: Emotion, attachment, trauma & neurobiology*. New York: Norton.

Winnicott, D.W. (1958). *Through Paediatrics to Psycho-Analysis: Collected papers*. London: Tavistock.

Wood, C. (1998). Lecture given to final year students of Art Therapy, Sheffield Centre for Psychotherapeutic Studies, Sheffield University, UK, June 1998.

Chapter 9

# Sandtray therapy
## A neurobiological approach

*Daniel S. Sweeney*

## Introduction

In this era of focusing on the etiology and treatment of mental health challenges in light of neurobiological considerations, clinicians are compelled to consider the rationale and implementation of interventions in light of the brain. The effect on the brain of child abuse is phenomenal. For example, in research of child subjects with PTSD, there is evidence of broad neuronal atrophy and diminished development (De Bellis and Zisk, 2014). With this being the case, therapists have a responsibility to honor not only developmental level, but also neurobiological realities. Creative arts interventions, as discussed in this book, look to do this. This chapter focuses on one of these, in the discussion of sandtray therapy.

## Sandtray therapy

Sandtray therapy is a projective and expressive therapy that has the impressive quality of being extraordinarily adaptable. It can incorporate a wide variety of theoretical and technical psychotherapeutic approaches. It can neurobiologically reach beyond cortical interventions (which may have limited efficacy with trauma issues), into limbic and midbrain areas, with its sensory and kinesthetic quality. It can be directive or non-directive, verbal or nonverbal, and can incorporate techniques from a variety of therapeutic approaches. This makes sandtray therapy a truly cross-theoretical intervention.

Homeyer and Sweeney (in press) assert that sandtray therapy is cross-theoretical, not atheoretical. Sandtray therapy interventions and techniques should always be theoretically based. Sweeney (2011a) asserted that theory is always important, but theory without technique is basically philosophy. At the same time, techniques may be quite valuable, but techniques without theory are reckless and could be damaging. Sweeney further asserted:

> All therapists are encouraged to ponder some questions regarding employing techniques: (a) Is the technique developmentally appropriate? [which presupposes that developmental capabilities are a key therapeutic consideration]; (b) What theory underlies the technique? [which presupposes that techniques

should be theory-based]; and (c) What is the therapeutic intent in employing a given technique? [which presupposes that having specific therapeutic intent is clinically and ethically important]

(2011a, p. 236)

The definition of sandtray therapy reflects the contention that it is a cross-theoretical approach. As such, it does not include theory-specific language. Adapted from Homeyer and Sweeney (2011), the following definition is offered: Sandtray therapy is an expressive and projective mode of psychotherapy involving the unfolding and processing of intra- and interpersonal issues through the use of specific sandtray materials as a nonverbal medium of communication, led by the client or therapist and facilitated by a trained therapist.

There are numerous approaches to sandtray therapy, which cannot be fully discussed in this short chapter. Note, however, the specific and intentional use of the term *sandtray* therapy, as opposed to *sand play* therapy. Sandtray therapy includes any theoretical and technical use of sandtray materials in the psychotherapeutic process. Sand play therapy is the well-defined Jungian approach to sandtray therapy. I fully endorse *sand play* therapy, but believe the distinction is an important one.

A brief look at history: In 1920, British paediatrician Margaret Lowenfeld (1993) developed an approach to working with children using miniature toys and a sandtray. She was looking for:

[a] medium which would in itself be instantly attractive to children and which would give them and the observer a language, as it were, through which communication could be established . . . if given the right tools, they would find their way to communication of their interior experience.

(p. 281)

She found that this approach worked with clients of all ages, noting that this approach was "welcomed by adult patients as an aid to their understanding of themselves and to communications with their therapist" (p. 5). As clients created their "worlds" in the sandtray, Lowenfeld's approach was named the World Technique.

## Benefits and rationale

Numerous benefits and rationales for the sandtray therapy process have been posited (Sweeney and Homeyer, 2009; Homeyer and Sweeney, 2011; Sweeney, 2011b):

- *Sandtray therapy gives expression to nonverbalized emotional issues.* Expressive and projective therapies provide a distinct language for clients unable or unwilling to verbalize. The sandtray process is the language, and

the miniatures are the words. Along with this, clients need no creative or artistic ability to participate.
- *Sandtray therapy has a unique kinesthetic quality.* There is a unique kinesthetic and sensory experience in sandtray therapy, which serves as an extension of foundational attachment needs.
- *Sandtray therapy serves to create a necessary therapeutic distance for clients.* When clients have difficulty expressing themselves through verbalization, they can do so through a projective medium such as sandtray therapy. Frequently, it is easier for traumatized clients to "speak" through sandtray miniatures than to directly verbalize pain.
- *This therapeutic distance that sandtray therapy provides creates a safe place for abreaction to occur.* Traumatized clients desperately need a therapeutic setting in which to abreact. The therapeutic distance provided by sandtray therapy creates a place where unexpressed issues can emerge and be safely relived, as well as the opportunity to experience the associated negative emotions.
- *Sandtray therapy is an effective intervention for traumatized clients.* The neurobiological effects of trauma (including prefrontal cortical dysfunction, overactivation of the limbic system, and deactivation of the Broca's area, part of the brain responsible for speech; van der Kolk, 2014) point to the benefit of nonverbal interventions. The apparent neurobiological inhibitions of cognitive processing and verbalization contend for an expressive intervention such as sandtray therapy.
- *Sandtray therapy is effective in overcoming client resistance.* The inherently engaging and nonthreatening nature of sandtray therapy often captivates the involuntary or reticent client. For clients who are resistant or fear verbal conflict, sandtray therapy can provide a safer means of engagement.
- *Sandtray therapy provides a needed and effective communication medium for the client with poor verbal skills.* It is always important to provide developmentally appropriate therapeutic interventions for child clients—in addition, there are clients who have poor verbal skills. Sandtray therapy helps clients who experience language deficits or delays, social difficulties or physiological challenges.
- *Conversely, sandtray therapy cuts through verbalization used as a defense.* For clients who are verbally astute, yet may be developmentally delayed or who use verbalization as a means to defend or manipulate, sandtray therapy provides a means of legitimate communication. Similarly, for clients who use rationalization and intellectualization as a defense, sandtray therapy can cut through these defenses.
- *The challenge of transference may be effectively addressed through sandtray therapy.* Sandtray therapy provides a cross-theoretical means for transference issues to be safely identified and addressed. In sandtray therapy, the miniatures and tray become the objects of transference or the means by which transference issues are identified and focused upon.

- *Finally, deeper intrapsychic issues are arguably accessed more thoroughly and more rapidly through sandtray therapy.* The aggregate benefits and rationales for sandtray therapy noted above create a therapeutic milieu where deep and complex intrapsychic and interpersonal issues can be safely approached. Many clients are psychologically and neurobiologically defended when addressing challenges to their injured psyche, and the safety of sandtray therapy can serve to decrease defenses and increase disclosure.

## Linkage to neurobiology

Sandtray therapy, like many expressive therapy interventions, impacts the psychology and neurobiology of clients and their presenting issues. Rather than the limited focus on the executive functioning of the cortical area of the brain, which has limited ability to process trauma (van der Kolk, 2014), sandtray creates an experiential, nonverbally based experience to process deeper neurobiological issues.

As other chapters in this book have mentioned, for clients to experience change, perhaps even reversal of the accumulated neural erosion of damaged attachment and trauma, interventions must target underdeveloped and corrupted regions of the brain (Perry, 2009). This is particularly important in the regions most impacted by trauma, including: relational connection, self-regulation, executive functioning, memory, and sensory integration. To resolve and reform dysfunctional neural networks, interventions must activate these systems (Perry, 2009; Gaskill and Perry, 2012, 2014). Perry summarizes this: "Matching the correct therapeutic activities to the specific developmental stage and physiological needs of a maltreated or traumatized child is a key to success" (2006: 29). Sandtray can provide this.

Badenoch and Kestly (2015) provide an important summary of the neurological benefits of play and sandtray experiences as they relate to trauma work:

> What most needs to change is the embodied subjective sense within the implicit memory, since that is what continues to come into the present, bringing perceptions, feelings and behaviors with it.... It appears that the neural nets holding implicit memory open to new information when two conditions are met: The implicit memory is alive in the body and it is met with what is called a disconfirming experience. That is, the implicit memory is met with an embodied experience of what was missing and needed at the time of the original event.... In the context of a play therapy relationship that is intent on being alive to the present moment, it is possible for these disconfirming experiences to unfold in the moment-to-moment relational interchange surrounding the arising of these implicit memories.
> 
> (pp. 528–9)

As noted earlier, Homeyer and Sweeney (2011) use the sandtray creation as a springboard for therapist–client interaction and discussion. This itself has neurological benefit. Badenoch (2008) encourages discussion of the tray's meaning with the client, stating that, "in terms of brain integration, talking about the tray at this stage can help foster connection between the hemispheres by adding words to the rich experience that has unfolded nonverbally" (p. 224). This *hemispherical* perspective is echoed by Siegel: "To have a coherent story, the drive of the left to tell a logical story must draw on the information from the right. If there is a blockage, as occurs in PTSD, then the narrative may be incoherent" (2003: 15).

Badenoch (2008) also suggests that it is helpful to inquire about the feeling of the tray, as opposed to looking for cognitive meaning: "We don't want to catalyze a leap from right- to left-hemisphere processes, but rather open the highway for the right to offer itself to the left" (p. 224). This is supported by Gaskill and Perry (2012), who assert that, as "neural activity is transmitted to higher, more complex areas (limbic and cortical), more intricate cognitive associations are made, allowing interpretation of the experience" (p. 33). This should be a reminder to sandtray therapists that interpretation should be left to the client, for both emotional and neurobiological purposes.

Sandtray therapy is particularly suited to the limbic and neocortical areas of brain development. In Perry's (2006) model of *sequential neurodevelopment and therapeutic activity* (p. 41), play therapy and storytelling—primary elements of sandtray therapy—are the primary therapeutic and enrichment activities for the limbic and cortical brain areas.

Traumatized clients need a soothing intervention. The trauma has left the client's brain in an alarm state, where alarm reactions trump cortical processing (Perry, 2006; van der Kolk, 2006, 2014). The cortex can be overwhelmed by lower regions of the brain, and thus an intervention such as sandtray therapy, which does not rely on verbal processing and executive functioning, helps to soothe clients who may have alarm reactions in the therapy process. Perry and Hambrick (as cited in Gaskill and Perry, 2012) emphasize that, "until state regulation or healthy homeostasis is established at the brainstem level, higher brain mediated treatments will be less effective" (p. 40).

In the *neurosequential model of therapeutics* developed by Perry (Perry, 2006, 2009; Gaskill and Perry, 2012, 2014), it is suggested that therapy with traumatized and neglected children—as well as adolescents and adults—begin with a focus on the lower brain regions (the brainstem and diencephalon (midbrain)) and work upwards. This would include moving through the higher brain areas identified by Perry as the limbic and cortical areas. Perry (2009) posits:

> Once there is improvement in self-regulation, the therapeutic work can move to more relational-related problems (limbic) using more traditional play or arts therapies; ultimately, once fundamental dyadic relational skills have improved, the therapeutic techniques can be more verbal and insight oriented (cortical) using any variety of cognitive-behavioral or psychodynamic approach.
>
> (p. 252)

Sandtray therapy follows this very progression. The initial therapeutic work, from the very first touching of the sand, is fundamentally brainstem and diencephalon related. Badenoch (2008) asserts that arranging the sand is anexperience that, "encourages vertical integration, linking body, limbic region, and cortex in the right hemisphere" (p. 223). This sand play focuses on the tactile, motor and attunement approaches needed for the brainstem—as well as the rhythm, simple narrative and physical warmth needed for the diencephalon (see Perry, 2006). Sandtray can then bring a client to the relational and narrative elements of play therapy needed for the limbic area, moving to the narrative and conversational (as well as insight) needed for the cortex (Perry, 2006).

The first chapter in this book discusses the "use-dependent" nature of the brain (Perry, 2006, 2009). Sandtray therapy honors this neurological reality. Perry (2009) notes that many clinical interventions target "the innervated cortical or limbic (i.e., cognitive and relational interactions) regions of the brain and not the innervating source of the dysregulation (lower stress-response networks)" (p. 244). Because sandtray begins with the basic materials of sand and miniatures, it begins with the lower stress-response networks, before moving on to cognitive and relational interactions through the processing of sandtray creations.

## Sandtray protocol and activities

The basic materials in sandtray therapy include one or more sandtrays, water (if possible—if only one tray is available, it should be a dry tray), and a selection of miniatures. There is no need to have an elaborate and expansive collection, which may in fact be overwhelming for some clients.

"Standard" sandtrays are usually $20 \times 30 \times 3$ inches, painted blue on the inside to simulate sky and water, and half-filled with quality sand. The tray size is significant—it intrinsically provides boundaries and limits for clients, and the sandtray creation can be viewed in a single glance. The height of the tray(s) should be at the average desktop level, preferably with some surface space around the base of the tray. Some clients prefer to place miniatures outside the tray, possibly to serve as issues that they are not ready to approach and process.

A selection of miniatures should be made available for use in the sandtray (see Homeyer and Sweeney (2011) for detail on categories of miniatures). These should be deliberately selected (not collected) exclusively for the sandtray therapy process. On average, a collection of 400–500 miniatures is satisfactory. Thousands of miniatures are not necessary (and may in fact be emotionally flooding for some clients).

Sandtray therapy protocol will vary according to therapeutic theory and style, but there are some basic elements detailed by Homeyer and Sweeney (2011) that I consider important in the overall process. These include: (1) room preparation, (2) introduction to the client, (3) creation of the sandtray, (4) post-creation process, (5) sandtray clean-up and (6) documenting the session. These are briefly discussed as follows.

## Room preparation

The therapist should ensure that the sandtray materials are in place, check that there no buried items in the tray, and ensure that the sand is somewhat flat. The miniatures should be arranged in an orderly and consistent manner. This creates an atmosphere of predictability and safety. The therapist should sit in a non-intrusive place, but remain fully involved—thus not invasive in the developing dynamic between the client and the media. The furniture in the room should facilitate client movement between the tray(s) and the collection of miniatures.

## Introduction to the client

The therapist may use a non-directive or directive approach. A non-directive approach involves giving very minimal directions to the client. This allows the creation to be entirely the result of the client's interaction with the miniatures, tray, and sand. A directive approach can be used when the therapist sees the need to address a specific issue, or may be necessary when clients are overwhelmed with a free and unstructured experience. Giving definitive instructions may feel more protective for these clients.

## Creation of the sandtray

The therapist should honor both the process and the product (scene). Kalff (1980) talked about the need to create a "free and protected" space. This involves the Jungian concept of *temenos*: that the therapy room and process—and the sandtray itself—provide a boundary between the sacred and the profane. Clients must believe they are fully safe—emotionally, psychologically, spiritually, and physically.

## Post-creation process

Some sandtray therapists prefer to allow the creative process and creation to stand alone, arguing that this in itself activates the client's internal healing process. These clinicians will thus not discuss or process the creation in the sandtray. Others will use the creative process and creations as a springboard for discussion and continued verbal and nonverbal work with the client. This is my common process, and I experience clients discovering insights regardless of whether it is a directed or non-directed experience.

## Sandtray clean-up

My perspective here is related to our work as play therapists. In play therapy, I view the play as the language and the toys as the words—in sandtray therapy, the miniatures are the words. Fundamentally, they are the expression of the client's emotional life and inner self. Thus, I do not want to communicate that the client's emotional expression needs to be "cleaned up" and is, therefore, unacceptable. Weinrib (1983) said, "To destroy a picture in the patient's presence would be to devalue a completed creation, to break the connection between the patient and his inner self, and the unspoken connection to the therapist" (p. 14).

## Documenting the sandtray session

Typically, photographs of the completed sandtray creations are taken and placed in the client file. This should be done with the client's permission. These pictures can be invaluable in reviewing the progress of clients over a period of time. Additionally, this photographic narrative can be reviewed by the therapist and client in the assessment of progress and evaluation for termination.

## Sandtray case examples

### Child

Adapted from a case discussed in Homeyer and Sweeney (2011), this case involves two girls (aged 6 and 8). It should first be noted that the following sandtray was not a part of the treatment plan. This case represents one session, in which sandtray therapy was utilized. The presenting issue was that the girls were having a challenging time adjusting (emotionally and behaviorally) to the current divorce process of their parents.

The treatment plan involved seeing the girls in sibling group play therapy (Sweeney *et al.*, 2014), while concurrently seeing the parents in filial therapy (Landreth and Bratton, 2006). A significant part of the parent intervention was to create a predictable parent–child experience in each home.

The sandtray therapy experience came about as a result of a scheduling misunderstanding. On a week when the parents were expected, for continued filial therapy training, the father brought the two girls in. Standard play therapy equipment was not available this week; however, sandtray therapy materials were.

The sandtray materials were introduced to the girls, and directive instructions were given. The girls were told: "On one side, build what your world was like before the divorce. On the other side, build what your world is like now." I was unsure if the girls could comprehend what was meant by the term world, but they were not inhibited.

The 8-year-old girl chose to divide the tray in half using tombstones. This was certainly a vivid depiction of the "death" of their parents' marriage. The metaphorical (arguably right-brained) display of the child's recognition of the permanence of the end of her parents' relationship was striking.

On the left side of the tray, there was a couple, with the female figure clearly leaning towards the male figure. The girls both described this as a representation of how their parents were always arguing and underscored that the leaning woman depicted how their mother was particularly loud and aggressive with her words.

On this side of the tray were also two girl figures in the lower portion of the left half, far from the adult figures and with their faces against the side of the tray. This displayed the girls' emotional and physical need to hide from their parents when they were fighting.

On the right side of the tray, the scene was divided in half with fences. As opposed to the thorough separation of the two sides of the tray—completely separated by the tombstones—the divisions of this side of the tray were somewhat open and porous. The state of child custody at the time was joint physical custody, and the girls often experienced their parents interacting.

The top half of the right side of the tray was their description of living with their mother. They chose a female figure in academic regalia, as they recognized the relationship between this figure and going to school, stating that their mother had recently gone back to school. They also noted that, between school and their mother's social life ("she's dating"), she didn't have time for the girls. Distinctly, the two figures they selected for themselves in this section of the tray were facing away from their mother. These figures were larger than all of the figures in the tray.

On the bottom half of this side, the girls are facing their father. The father was noted to be more relational in the filial therapy process. However, the girls selected a judge figure for their father and did not discuss this selection. It is possible that this represented some part of their perception of their father—or, with the custody issue not finally resolved at this point, it could have represented their awareness of the judge's power in this process.

Although this was not an ongoing sandtray therapy case, the vivid depiction of the girls' perception of the divorce and relationship dynamics is an example of the therapeutic power of sandtray therapy. The majority of the benefits and rationale of sandtray therapy noted earlier in the chapter can be seen in this singular exercise.

## *Adolescent*

Adapted from a case discussed in Sweeney (2011b), this case involves a 14-year-old boy, Rand (name changed, for privacy reasons), who was referred for counseling by his parents. Rand was reported as being noncompliant with his parents, having conflict with his peers and siblings, and arguing with teachers at school. It was noted that his parents were experiencing couple conflict, to which an undetermined amount of Rand's behavior could be attributed. Although the parents were offered a counseling referral, they firmly declined.

At the beginning of the therapy process, Rand was invited to create several sandtrays with minimal directions. He appeared to enjoy the activity, but little therapeutic material emerged. A couple of sessions following this, a solution-focused intervention was employed, using the "miracle question." With preadolescents and adolescents, the wording is occasionally changed from "miracle" to "magic." Although most adolescents understand the word "miracle," my experience has been that there is often a better response to "magic." In this case, the following instructions were given:

> I'd like to ask you to do something specific in the sand tray today, Rand. I've got a question for you to consider, and then make a scene in the tray. If something magical were to happen tonight, while you were sleeping, and tomorrow morning you woke up, and all this stuff we've been talking about was gone – pretty nice if we had that kind of magic, huh? – what would it look like in the morning? Could you make a scene in the tray about what this would look like?
>
> (Sweeney, 2011b: 71)

Rand went to work right away, quickly dividing the tray in half, using trees and fences to separate the sides. Without further instruction from the therapist, he created a scene about how he viewed things in his "world" currently, and how he would like things to be if something magical could actually happen. These specific instructions were not given, but Rand took the process where he wanted to go.

On the side of the sand tray that characterized how Rand viewed the problem at the time, there were multiple scenes of conflict, each one involving himself. These included conflicts at school and at home. Interestingly, on this side of the tray, Rand chose only animals. This may be a representation of the therapeutic distance discussed earlier that can be created in sandtray therapy. It was not surprising that it was a challenge for Rand to identify with his problematic behavior. He was, however, willing and able to take a measure of responsibility for his disruptive behavior, as this was the first tray (or verbal expression) in which he identified his challenging behavior—in this case calling himself a "trouble maker."

The opposite side of the tray represented the focus of the solution-focused miracle question. Here, Rand was able to initially consider a future apart from the presenting problem. Interestingly, he did not include himself on this side of the tray. It is a common inquiry in processing a tray whether or not clients have placed themselves in the tray. On this side of the tray, Rand included his parents. In contrast to the animals on the other side of the tray, he selected human figures (one female and one male) and placed them in a setting that Rand identified as "paradise." He expressed some sadness about how much his parents argued and stated that he wished they could find a "magic place where there were no fights."

Rand himself acknowledged that a significant part of the source of his disruptive problems related to his parents' conflict. He wasn't blaming his parents and did not directly attribute his own disruptive behavior to them—at least not at a verbal or conscious level. When asked about why he did not include himself on the "paradise" side of the tray, Rand said that he did not want his "problems" to get in the way of their happiness. There was sadness in his voice and facial expression as he made this point.

The creation and processing of this tray represented a turning point in the therapeutic process. Rand's disruptive behaviors began to decrease, but, more significantly, his parents agreed to seek couple counseling. After this began (with positive results), Rand's noncompliance subsided considerably.

## Adult

This case involves the final sandtray creation of an adult who was in therapy regarding the stresses of working through a graduate academic program. There were a minimal number of miniatures chosen for this tray, but the client (Marion; name changed, for privacy reasons) was deeply impacted by the therapeutic journey and this final sandtray. With Marion's permission, the following is a direct transcript of the client's journal of her final tray. She titled the tray: "The journey."

> For my expression in "The journey," I chose the octopus, the scorpion, the sword, the little girl behind the wall, the cross, and the graduate.
>
> The octopus was a representation of my feeling somewhat "all over the place." One arm busy doing one thing, another doing something else and the others doing work – involving my graduate internship, being a mother, nurse, housekeeper, gardener, vet, chauffeur, wife, disciplinarian, writer, daughter, sister, bookkeeper, and (oh my gosh) did I mention graduate student? WOW! I feel floppy and sometimes with no bones to hold me up, out of control more than ever at times.
>
> The scorpion was a representation of feeling poisoned and stabbed by some of my perceptions of what I feel I am as a graduate student. Very different than most, I'm sure! I was very hard on myself. I feel I lost complete track of my inner child. I have never been more serious about life. (I have always been in touch with my inner child in the past.)
>
> As someone said to me early on . . . meant as a compliment . . . "You are not what I consider a graduate student, but a mom going to graduate school." So, I basically contorted and morphed into having new perspectives of my life and busy adjusting to it.
>
> The cross and the sword have been my means of survival and sanity through this incredible journey. If these weren't available, I don't think I would have made it this far. God has provided a sense of confidence and assurance for my decisions related to the journey. The sword represents a fighting spirit that I believe God provided me to fight off negative feelings, disbelief, guilt and THE SCORPION!
>
> As the graduate stands high up on the hill in the sand, I feel there's still a bit of a journey which includes finishing my thesis, interviews, getting a job and paying back student loans. YIKES! Not to mention . . . getting back in touch with the little girl behind the wall. I'm really looking forward to that!!!

This sandtray experience put the entire therapeutic journey into perspective for Marion. She was able to get in touch with deep issues, as well as summarize the therapeutic process. The recognition of the amount of energy that she was placing into each role (represented by the octopus tentacles) helped Marion realize the extent of her stress, and the need to develop a self-care plan. Additionally, she recognized—for the first time—that there was a level of vicarious traumatization that she was already experiencing as a mental health therapist in training. With every sandtray creation Marion made, she experienced (in her own words) "deep emotional release".

## Conclusion

A major element in sandtray therapy is to provide clients with a safe place to tell their story. With regard to safety, van der Kolk (2002) argues that trauma always involves speechless terror—that traumatized clients are basically unable to put feelings into words and are thus left with intense emotions that can't be fully verbalized. He also states that, as long as clients "are unable to talk about their traumatic experiences, they simply have no story, and instead, the trauma is likely to be expressed as an embodiment of what happened" (2003: 311).

Owing to its incredibly adaptive and flexible nature, sandtray therapy has many psychotherapeutic applications. Its deep intrapsychic and interpersonal nature touches clients in profound ways. It is truly cross-theoretical and can be nondirective or directive, and almost any treatment technique can be adapted for use in sandtray therapy. Having made these assertions, I would argue that traumatized clients are not healed through the use of techniques. People experience healing through process and relationship. This can and does occur through sandtray therapy.

This focus on relationship has both psychological and neurobiological benefits. Perry and Pate (1994) appropriately state:

> It is the 'relationship' which enables access to parts of the brain involved in social affiliation, attachment, arousal, affect, anxiety regulation and physiological hyper-reactivity. Therefore, the elements of therapy which induce positive changes will be the relationship and the ability of the child to re-experience traumatic events in the context of a safe and supportive relationship.
>
> (p. 142)

## Key points

- Sandtray therapy is explained as a cross-theoretical creative arts psychotherapy with nonverbal, sensory, and kinesthetic qualities.
- Sandtray therapy is defined as "an expressive and projective mode of psychotherapy involving the unfolding and processing of intra- and interpersonal

issues through the use of specific sandtray materials as a nonverbal medium of communication, led by the client or therapist and facilitated by a trained therapist."
- The chapter identifies nine specific rationales for the employment of sandtray therapy.
- The neurobiological benefits for the use of sandtray therapy are summarized, focused on its use as a nonverbal intervention for traumatized clients who have limited access to executive function and verbalizing areas of the brain, while also experiencing considerable activity in the limbic system.
- Basic sandtray therapy materials and a basic therapeutic protocol involving six fundamental considerations are summarized.
- Three case studies are presented—with a child, an adolescent, and an adult.

## References

Badenoch, B. (2008). *Being a Brain-wise Therapist: A practical guide to interpersonal neurobiology*. New York: W.W. Norton.

Badenoch, B., and Kestly, T. (2015). Exploring the neuroscience of healing play at every age. In D. Crenshaw and A. Stewart (eds) *Play Therapy: A comprehensive guide to theory and practice* (pp. 524–38). New York: Guilford Press.

De Bellis, M., and Zisk, A. (2014). The biological effects of childhood trauma. *Child & Adolescent Psychiatric Clinics of North America, 23*(2), 185–222.

Gaskill, R., and Perry, B. (2012). Child sexual abuse, traumatic experiences, and their impact on the developing brain. In P. Goodyear-Brown (ed.) *Handbook of Child Sexual Abuse: Identification, assessment and treatment* (pp. 29–48). Hoboken, NJ: Wiley.

Gaskill, R., and Perry, B. (2014). The neurobiological power of play: Using the neurosequential model of therapeutics to guide play in the healing process. In C. Malchiodi and D. Crenshaw (eds) *Creative Arts and Play Therapy for Attachment Problems* (pp. 178–96). New York: Guilford Press.

Homeyer, L., and Sweeney, D. (2011). *Sandtray Therapy: A practical manual*. (2nd edn). New York: Routledge.

Homeyer, L., and Sweeney, D. (in press). Sandtray Therapy: A variety of approaches. In B. Turner (ed.) *The International Handbook of Sandplay Therapy*. New York: Routledge.

Kalff, D. (1980). *Sandplay, a Psychotherapeutic Approach to the Psyche*. Santa Monica, CA: Sigo Press.

Landreth, G., and Bratton, S. (2006). *Child Parent Relationship Therapy (CPRT): A 10-session filial therapy model*. New York: Routledge.

Lowenfeld, M. (1993). *Understanding Children's Sandplay: The world technique*. Chippenham, UK: Rowe. (Originally published as *The World Technique*, George Allen & Unwin, 1979)

Perry, B. (2006). Applying principles of neurodevelopment to clinical work with maltreated and traumatized children: The neurosequential model therapeutics. In N.B. Webb (ed.) *Working with Traumatized Youth in Child Welfare* (pp. 27–52). New York: Guilford Press.

Perry, B. (2009). Examining child maltreatment through a neurodevelopmental lens: Clinical applications of the neurosequential model of therapeutics. *Journal of Loss and Trauma*, *14*, 240–55.

Perry, B., and Pate, J. (1994). Neurodevelopment and the psychobiological roots of post-traumatic stress disorder. In L. Koziol and C. Stout (eds) *The Neuropsychology of Mental Disorders: A practical guide* (pp. 129–46). Springfield, IL: Charles C. Thomas.

Siegel, D. (2003). An interpersonal neurobiology of psychotherapy: The developing mind and the resolution of trauma. In D. Siegel and M. Solomon (eds) *Healing Trauma: Attachment, mind, body and brain* (pp. 1–56). New York: W.W. Norton.

Sweeney, D. (2011a). Group play therapy. In C.E. Schaefer (ed.) *Foundations of Play Therapy* (2nd edn, pp. 227–52). New York: Wiley.

Sweeney, D. (2011b). Integration of sandtray therapy and solution-focused techniques for treating noncompliant youth. In A. Drewes, S. Bratton and C. Schaefer (eds) *Integrative Play Therapy* (pp. 61–74). New York: John Wiley.

Sweeney, D., and Homeyer, L. (2009). Sandtray therapy. In A. Drewes (ed.) *Blending of Play Therapy and Cognitive Behavioral Therapy* (pp. 297–318). New York: Wiley.

Sweeney, D., Baggerly, J., and Ray, D. (2014). *Group Play Therapy: A dynamic approach*. New York: Routledge.

van der Kolk, B. (2002). In terror's grip: Healing the ravages of trauma. *Cerebrum*, *4*, 34–50.

van der Kolk, B. (2003). The neurobiology of trauma and abuse. *Child & Adolescent Psychiatric Clinics of North America*, *12*, 293–317.

van der Kolk, B. (2006). Clinical implications of neuroscience research in PTSD. *Annals of the New York Academy of Science*, *1071*(IV), 277–93.

van der Kolk, B. (2014). *The Body Keeps the Score: Brain, mind, and body in the healing of trauma*. New York: Penguin.

Weinrib, E. (1983). *Images of Self: The sandplay therapy process*. Boston, MA: Sigo Press.

Chapter 10

# Telling tales
## Weaving new neural networks

*Aideen Taylor de Faoite, Eileeen Prendiville and Theresa Fraser*

Storytelling has been a part of human existence since we developed the capacity to communicate; our ability to tell a story contributes to making us human. Stories reflect the wisdom of time, from the first early drawings on the cave wall, to the writings of the Egyptians, to the retelling of myths and legends. Stories have been used to recollect heroic events and to understand tragedy. Campfire stories are told to calm fears and doubts. There are stories in all cultures to explain creation, to account for the trickster, to recount epic journeys and the overcoming of obstacles. Stories have been told to share values and traditions, to teach and share insights and to entertain. They can be factual or fanciful, personal or cultural. In many traditions, the storyteller has a special place, as the wise man, the person who provides spiritual guidance or the healer.

In this chapter, we explore how stories can be used within creative psychotherapeutic interventions in a neurobiological and neurosequential model, in particular focusing on their value for working with the limbic and cortical systems and integrating the left and right hemispheres of the brain. We consider the role of storytelling in human development and the development of narrative in play, placing these interventions in the theoretical framework of narrative theory, therapy and social constructionism.

## The place of storytelling within therapeutic practice

The 6 Rs identified by Perry (see Chapter 2) are an integral part of the planning and implementation of storytelling and narrative in therapy. A safe, fear-free space is created, with the therapist initially as empathetic audience and the client as the storyteller; this establishes the context of the *relationship* and activation of the bonding system. As a basic human endeavour, storytelling is appropriate across all stages of development. The developmental stage, however, becomes important in the methods used to tell or elicit the story. Pictures, props and enactment may be more appropriate for a younger client, whereas writing, art and spoken word may be more *relevant* for a more developmentally mature client. The use of different media allows for the *repetition* of stories. The client can choose to tell their story through play and enactment, through sand play and drawing or writing. As adults, we are also often drawn back to re-read a story. The initial joy of discovering the story can be revisited and is *rewarding*. The stucture of a story (with a beginning, a middle and an end) provides *rhythm*. The story begins in a certain space and time and is brought back to the present with its end. Owing to the breadth of stories available, whether factual or fanciful, *respect* can be paid to the client, their family and their culture.

Therapy is about relationships and storytelling, and the tradition of storytelling and its contribution to human development can be seen in a number of theoretical models and approaches in psychotherapy. In play therapy, the child tells a story through their play, including enactments, sand play and the pictures they create. Such stories can be wordless (storytelling precedes language), indicating the predominant involvement of the right hemisphere, or accompanied by language, indicating the involvement of the left hemisphere. The parallel use of play supports the integration of both hemispheres. In narrative therapy, the adult tells a story about their life, their worries and stresses, interactions and relationships. Their story in therapy may be a different story from that told to friends and family. The storyteller decides where the story starts and ends and what obstacles have to be overcome within the tale. There is the story that brings the individual to therapy and the stories told as they progress and as they reach resolution. There is the story a person tells about themselves, the story a person perceives the community tells about them and the story about the influence other people's stories might have. In the context of therapy, the story acts as a container. The use of storytelling and narrative in therapy is a collaborative process that supports the client as expert on their own life. The client can choose the predominant story that they wish to share at any particular time.

Children's play and storytelling often reflect their life experiences, and this play supports emotional health and well-being (Howard and McInnes, 2012). The language and storying in children's everyday play can reflect specific experiences of traumatic events (Bateman *et al.*, 2013a, 2013b, 2015). In a therapeutic context, storytelling, narrative and writing can emerge spontaneaously, or they can be introduced by the therapist. Spontaneous stories emerge from the child's play when a safe environment is created to support the child to play with a range of toys. In the play therapy room, the child may choose to play with the doll's house, enact familiar roles in the kitchen or create a picture in the sand using the miniatures. Such stories open a window into the child's internal world and give clues about their world-view and embodied memories. Children may voice a story as they play or they may be invited to tell the story afterward. The child may be invited to draw a picture, for example, a person, a house and a tree, and tell the story of their picture. To facilitate the elaboration of the story, and allow for progression from the right hemishere to the left and back again to support neural integration, the child may be invited to think about where the tree is. For example, is it in a field, in a forest, growing through an old house? How did it get there? What does it think about/feel about where it is? How old is it? What has happened to it in the past? What might happen in the future? This can then be told back to the child as a meta-story of the tree, beginning with, 'Once upon a time a long time ago' or 'Not so long ago', and ending with, 'the end' or 'to be continued', depending on the context.

Storytelling can be incorporated into therapy using techniques such as bibliotherapy, life-story work and therapeutic storytelling. Storytelling introduces metaphors to therapy, either as a metaphor in the story or the use of story as a metaphor for the problem. Metaphors allow for distancing from emotionally laden issues (Sunderland, 2006). Stories are engaging and motivating. Stories help to make coherent an otherwise seemingly random sequence of events. The structure of a story is important, with a beginning and an end and, in the middle, an obstacle to be overcome and perhaps people or objects that are there to help. The roles of storyteller and audience also provide a predictability that is supportive to clients who have experienced trauma and provide a social context. Engagement in a story helps to bypass defences and resistance, while allowing for identification with the protagonist. Endings are not fixed and can be changed. This flexibility in stories allows the client to try out endings that might be different to their experience, without having to experience the consequences of such actions in the real world. Just as in play, where children can try on and try out roles, relationships and the consequences of action within a safe space (Howard and McInnes, 2013), the trying out of different stories, different characters and different endings in the imagination can in turn be a catalyst for change or catharsis.

The development of narrative skills, play and storytelling is interdependent. Initially, storytelling is nonverbal: it is our way of making sense of our experiences and our environment. We think in images, experience the here and now in an embodied way (all sensory input enters through the lower parts of the brain), develop implicit memories and working models wordlessly (Damasio, 1999) and later apply words (shared symbols) to this process. The spiral of play (Kestly, 2015), the progression to narrative and the interweaving of play and story, supports collaboration between the right and left hemispheres of the brain by developing neural pathways and facilitates the integration of novel or confusing experiences. Narrative skills are often acquired in play, with the support of an adult. This happens from an early age, when the adult provides a running commentary on what the child is doing or looking at in the environment. For example, the mother of a young baby might notice how they are drawn to the movement of leaves on the trees and comment, 'You are looking at the trees, you're noticing how the light is coming through the leaves'. This narrative might continue until the baby's attention is drawn elsewhere. The development of narrative continues with the child beginning to interact with objects and using them 'as if' they are something else. For example, when a child first picks up a block and says hello, 'as if' they were on a mobile phone, the adult might comment on who the child is talking to on the phone, and so the story and play develop. As well as through commentary, Trevarthen (1995) suggests that narrative skills are facilitated by the mother or primary caregiver in their interaction with the child when singing traditional rhymes and songs. These include skills of build-up, climax and resolution.

Bruner and Lucariello (1989) propose that stories emerge between 22 and 36 months and identify how these stories become more structured and complex over time. They argue that the purpose of these stories is often to recreate the inner child's world and to solve problems. Nicolopoulou (2006) suggests that, although play and narrative skills initially develop independently, they soon become interdependent. Initially in play, focus is on the representation of the character. As the child acts in role, they gain clarity as to the character's motivations, desires and belief. This, in turn, facilitates the development of a more comprehensive plot. The play extends the storytelling, and storytelling extends the play.

Narrative play therapy brings together the developmental potential of play and narrative and the theories of narrative therapy and social constructionism (Taylor de Faoite, 2011). Narrative theory assumes that people's actions are guided by culturally diverse meanings and the stories that they continuously construct about themselves (Smith, 1997). Constructionists believe that the concept of the Self is a social construction. The person is identified as an active agent engaged in intentional activity. The person is situated in a culture, a social setting and relationships. Stories are seen as the means by which we express ourselves and these relationships. The role of the therapist is to create a safe space to allow stories to emerge in the context of the therapeutic relationship. This space is created in the presentation of the physical environment, the emotional tone and the therapist's presence. A 'curious but not knowing' stance is adopted by the therapist. Boundaries, roles and responsibilities are communicated by the therapist. When working with a child client, the role of the therapist is to play alongside them and record their stories. The therapist may also have a role as storyteller, retelling the child's dictated stories or identifying stories that might be supportive and helpful to the child. In listening to the stories told by their clients, a therapist may initially be confused. Through conversation and questioning, the story is reconstructed. Questioning can be used to support construction of the story in a comprehensive manner, finding a beginning, a middle and an end (Taylor de Faoite, 2011).

Storying can be written as well as verbal. Writing a journal can be a useful way of exploring and externalizing our life stories and a means of organizing experiences. In writing stories down, the individual can begin to see how stories and thoughts can influence our feelings and behaviours. When we realize this, we can make choices to accept or change these stories. Bolton (1999) highlights the value of writing to help people find an order in the chaos, muddle and distress of their daily life, with stories being written and rewritten with different endings and different voices. The writing process allows the individual to think about different aspects of the self and allows them to pay attention to what is fruitful for them. Pennebaker (2000) has explored the use of writing as a way of increasing physical and emotional well-being. In his research, participants were asked to write about a traumatic experience for 15 minutes a day, for 5 weeks. A number of health, social and academic benefits were noted. Participants visited the doctor less, reported that they were happier and had more positive social interactions. Others have explored how writing about something for which we are grateful can impact on our happiness and well-being. After a 10-week intervention that involved writing about events for which they were grateful, Eammons and McCullough (2003) found that participants were more optimistic and felt better about their lives. They were more able to garnish support from others, had more positive interactions, slept better and exercised more.

## Stories and neurosequential therapy

Brain development hinges on a complex interplay between the genes you are born with and the experiences you have (Shore, 1997). Individual working models, which impact on our expectations and our responses when faced with similar sensory experiences in the future, develop in response to recurring experience (Perry, 2001). Use-dependent neurons and neural systems are designed to develop and change in response to repeated and co-occuring experiences. Development is sequential and is rapid in early childhood.

Secure attachments support intellectual development, good relationships with others, respect by peers and good emotional regulation (Siegel, 2010). Although neuroscience does not specifically study the effect of attachment on brain development, the behaviours observed in a securely attached child parallel the function of the middle prefrontal cortex. These include good bodily regulation, attunement to others, emotional balance, ability to respond flexibly, fear modulation, empathy and insight (Siegel, 2010). 'By three years of age, the brain of the child is two and a half times more active than the brain of an adult and stays that way through the first decade of life' (Shore, 1997: 21).

Perry states that, 'the degree of brain plasticity is related to stage of development and area or system in the brain, for some brain areas such as the cortex, significant plasticity remains throughout life' (2006: 43). We can address unmet physiological and developmental needs with specific therapeutic activities. The aim of such interventions is to support the individual in overcoming adversity and reaching their potential. Intentional, patterned and repetitive neural activation will be required if reorganization (changes in the structure of the brain) is to occur (Perry and Szalavitz, 2006). In using knowledge of neurosequential development to underpin treatment planning, the aim is to target interventions at both the appropriate level and appropriate brain region.

Therapeutic enrichment activities for the cortex include storytelling and drama, as well as opportunities that help with making sense of experiences using cognitive behavioural approaches or other insight-oriented interventions. Narrative, storytelling and journaling are associated with the higher function areas of the brain – the limbic and cortical areas. Choosing an intervention at this level assumes either that interventions have already targeted the lower brain regions or that the development of previous systems in the sequence has not been compromised. If this is not the case, the play therapist might first introduce rhythmical activities to support somatosensory integration and improve links between higher and lower brain regions. Later, the focus can shift to addressing relational problems (limbic region) using more traditional play and art therapies.

The limbic system is associated with the mammalian brain or the emotional brain (Sunderland, 2006). This system lies between the reptilian brain, including the spinal cord and the brainstem, which is responsible for basic survival, including the fight, flight or freeze response, and the cortical system. The limbic system has a role in managing the fight or flight impulse. The emotions that activate this part of the brain include rage, fear, separation distress, caring and nurturing, social bonding, playfulness and explorative urges, and lust in adults (Panksepp, 1998). The primary developmental goal when the limbic system is organizing (the period of most active growth is between 1 and 4 years) is to have experiences that practise emotional regulation, empathy, affiliation and tolerance. Optimizing experiences include social experiences, narrative opportunities and complex movement. Beneficial therapeutic enrichment activities could include play and play therapy, opportunities for parallel play, as well as creative art activities and performing arts activities (Perry, 2006).

Experiences trigger a range of emotions in the limbic area. The child's understanding of these feelings and subsequent skills to regulate these feelings are enhanced by the presence of a supportive adult. Repeated experiences will result in strong neural connections that result in the firing of all elements of the neural connections. The limbic and cortical systems are supported by therapeutic interventions using storytelling and narrative. Siegel and Bryson (2011) suggest the strategy of 'name it to tame it' as a strategy to support the development of the limbic system. This includes naming and acknowledging the child's feelings. The parent provides a narrative of what has happened and names the feelings the child is experiencing. For example, when Aideen's daughter was a toddler, a bird flew into the house, eliciting feelings of surprise and fear. Using wordless storytelling (Damasio, 1999), she immediately enacted this experience where she used an object and flew it around the house and pretended to let it out of the window. She then wanted the story told at bedtime. The addition of language moved the experience more fully to the cortical region and enabled the story to become more elaborate and include naming and mastering the feelings of shock, surprise and the ultimate relief when the bird escaped out the window. The repetition of the narrative of a negative or positive experience supports neurological development. Telling the story helps develop links between the lower limbic system and the higher structures of the cortical system. In addition, the linkage of the story with imagery and/or metaphors engages both brain hemispheres, supports integration and transformation through enhanced understanding and builds vital structures that equip the person for both academic and relational success.

When relationship skills are established, therapeutic techniques can become more insight-oriented (neocortical region) using a variety of therapeutic approaches targeting the cortex (Perry and Hambrick, 2008: 42). Neuroscience has revealed that storytelling is a natural function of the brain. Damasio (1999) 'talked about the naturalness of wordless storytelling' and that this 'is inherent in the brain's tendency to select, sort, assemble and integrate the objects that it encounters in the environment' (as cited in Kestly, 2015: 161).

Storytelling and the development of coherent narrative play a key role in the integration of the left and right hemispheres. The left hemisphere of the brain is responsible for processing language. It is logical, literal and linear (Mills and Crowley 1986; Siegel, 2012). The left hemisphere likes to arrange all the individual puzzle pieces in the correct order. The right brain is holistic and nonverbal and likes to consider the big picture, including the meaning and feelings associated with an experience. The right hemisphere perceives the whole picture. Metaphors appear to be the language of the right hemisphere (Mills and Crowley, 1986) and autobiographical memory. By using storytelling therapeutically, the therapist facilitates the integration of the logical, linear left with the holistic, emotional right hemisphere of the brain.

The cortical system supports higher thinking functions, such as reasoning, reflecting, problem-solving, creativity and imagination. It is also involved in self-awareness, kindness, empathy and concern (Sunderland, 2006). Between the ages of 3 and 6 years (the most active growth stage for the cortex), the primary developmental goals are to develop creativity and respect, build a moral and spiritual foundation, as well as provide opportunities to practise abstract reasoning. Perry (2006) suggests that the organizing experiences that support these outcomes include social interactions, exploratory play, complex conversations, 'solitude, satiety and security' (p. 41).

Thanks to its hierarchical structure, the cortical system has a role in managing lower-functioning structures of the brain. The stories that emerge in the child's play support creativity and imagination and the development of problem-solving skills. Interactve play and questioning (e.g. 'What will happen next? What will we use instead?') support cortical functioning. Taking different perspectives and wondering what it might be like to be another character in the story help to develop empathy and concern. The process of telling one's story, whether a projected story or the child's life story, develops self-awareness. The repetition of stories, whether told or enacted, allows for the development of neural connections, thus changing the structure of the brain. This can be seen in the child's wish for special stories to be read over and over or in the reciting of a favourite poem. Quentin Blake's poem *All Join In* (1990) was a favourite in Aideen's household. It reflected the chaos of a busy household while introducing humour into interactions in the family. A favourite game was to add what was happening in the house at the time and jokingly invite everyone to 'all join in'.

## Child client

Amy was the older child of Barbara and John. John died tragically in a car accident close to the family home, when Amy was 18 months old and her brother was 6 months old. On the night of the accident, Barbara heard the sound of emergency vehicles before the police called to the house while she was reading Amy a bedtime story.

Prior to her father's sudden death, Amy was a happy, playful child, with a settled routine and good relationships with both parents. However, in the year following this, she became very clingy, and her sleep became unsettled. She presented for play therapy when 30 months old.

An intake meeting with Barbara was conducted, and a contract for six sessions of play therapy was agreed. Owing to Amy's young age, 45-minute sessions were scheduled. The sessions would be child-led, at least initially, and the therapist would provide a running commentary interspersed with silence. A large blue cloth defined the play space, within a general-purpose room in a local centre. A tray of sand and various toys, sorted into categories, were placed around the edges of the play mat in shallow, open boxes and cloth bags. A sensory bag included play-dough, scents and materials of different textures. A nurture bag included a baby doll, nappies, clothes, wipes, lotions and creams, a baby bottle and a dummy. It was agreed that Amy could choose if her mother accompanied her to the play room or waited outside the door. When the sessions took place, Amy wanted Barbara in the room and on the play mat for the first session, to sit and watch from a chair in the second, and stay outside the room with the door open by the third.

In the first session, Amy invited her mother on to the mat and began playing with the play-dough. Barbara had been coached to follow Amy's lead and occasionally provide some running commentary. Her mother began mirroring what Amy was doing with the dough. The therapist added some descriptive commentary to support and encourage Barbara. Barbara began to comment on the colour she chose and to describe Amy's actions with the play-dough, such as 'rolling, squeezing' etc. Amy explored the sensory nature of the dough with interest. Occasionally, Amy would look at the box beside her, and I commented on how she noticed the different toys. Towards the end of the first session, Amy began to explore the animal box, picking up an animal, looking at it and naming it. Amy quickly explored different boxes of toys, choosing a number of miniatures to play with. These included the furniture for the doll's house, some adults and children, a dog, a car and traffic lights that could be changed by moving a lever. She spent some time organizing different rooms with their suites of furniture. Each room was set up on a carpet tile beside the playmat. At the end of the session, she invited her mother to look at her creations, which seemed to represent domestic bliss.

The following three sessions, the different rooms were set up on the carpet tiles again, and Amy engaged in play with cars, the traffic lights, police, firemen, an adult and a little girl. This play appeared to be a re-enactment of the night of the accident. Scenes included the car crashing into the traffic lights and the fireman arriving. A different, more frenetic, energy level was noted during this play.

The last two sessions were marked by the introduction of a nurse character who came between the fireman and the child and drove off on a green light. At this stage, the rooms from the house moved on to the playmat. Amy then began playing with the nurture bag in typical mummies-and-babies doll play, where the doll was cared for, fed, changed and played with. This ended the contracted number of sessions. A natural break occurred, with the family going on holiday. Amy was offered the option of asking her mum if she wished to come back for two more sessions after their holiday. Barbara phoned to report that Amy had settled well into crèche after the holiday and was sleeping well. Amy never requested any further play therapy.

In reflecting on this case, it was clear that Amy had very positive early experiences that had allowed for a smooth integration of brain development. When she experienced the trauma of the death of her father, she was able to use earlier strategies to support her well-being and development. She was able to use therapy at the limbic and subcortical levels of brain functioning to understand and story her implicit memories. The three stages of therapy identified by Anne Bannister, namely reassurance, re-enactment and rehearsal, are apparent in this intervention. Initially, reassurance was established by the plan for Amy's mother to be close and the co-facilitation of the initial session. The range of miniatures available allowed Amy to enact her immature understanding of the accident and the arrival of the police to break the news to her mother. Rehearsal of the future and the integration of the real and the imagined were observed as the child moved the doll's house furniture from the not-playing space on the carpet to the playmat. This allowed for the nurse to get 'the green light' and the onset of nurture play. The atmosphere had moved from unease, to intensive action when the car crash was being re-enacted, to calm as the nurse drove off and the return of typical doll play. Amy was able to use play to narrate her story from her point of view. This was possible owing her easy temperament and her early experiences that had helped her develop emotional regulation.

## Adolescent client

Sean is the younger child of Mary and John. Both parents had significant alcohol and drug problems. Sean was taken into care as a toddler owing to neglect and a significant failure to thrive. Following a number of unsuccessful attempts to support Mary's rehabilitation, Sean was placed in long-term foster care and he settled into family life.

Sean was seen for twelve sessions of play therapy when he was 8 years old. As he moved into adolescence, his behaviour became more challenging for his foster family, and he was re-referred at age 13. It was hypothesized that Sean might be struggling to understand his early life experiences from his perspective as an adolescent.

Materials provided included sand, miniatures, paints and games. Sean initially explored the sand play tray but then engaged in several games of soccer. The therapist was assigned the role of the 'goalie', and Sean played the role of the 'skilled soccer player'. Sometimes, the rules were changed. Themes of what it was like to be a winner or a loser were explored, along with success and skill. The therapist held a curious stance and questioned and encouraged Sean to explore identity issues.

As it happened, the therapist had been involved in making a documentary, independent of her work as a therapist. This documentary followed a home birth, and Sean had seen a rerun of the programme on television the night before a therapy session. When he arrived at the session, Sean was excited to tell the therapist the news that he had seen the therapist on television. This was followed by extensive conversations about babies and mothers and their relationships. Sean's questioning indicated that he was struggling with why people had babies. He was curious about how babies are looked after and how they get their needs met. This conversation carried on over a number of sessions. Sean posed questions that helped him to develop a coherent picture of a mother's role. Although life-story work had been done with Sean previously, it appeared from Sean's questioning that he wished to understand what should happen, rather than what had happened to him as a baby. These conversations allowed Sean to understand the needs of babies, from having their basic needs met to experiencing safety and building relationships. Through this narrative process of questioning, wondering and collaboration, Sean was able to develop a more preferred identity of the skilled winner and a coherent narrative about how early experience should be and how babies should be looked after. The process of the repetition of the football game, with the ball going back and forwards between the therapist and client, allowed for the development of a relationship. The fact that, at 13–14 years old, Sean chose to play football reflected the flexibility of play and narrative in meeting the child's developmental needs. Physical activity soothes the body and promotes production of dopamine and seratonin. Cortical engagment is enhanced by simultaneous engagement in motor activity. The football game allowed for lots of repetition and a rhythm to develop, thus strengthening the development of neural networks. The interaction appeared to have been rewarding. Sean's foster parent reported that Sean was always ready on time for therapy and enjoyed coming. The safe environment created in therapy allowed Sean to develop a coherent narrative about what family life should be like, without being critical or judging in any way his family of origin. When answering questions posed by Sean, the therapist was respectful to his family and culture. Sean was facilitated in writing his preferred, future-oriented story.

## Adult client

Irena had engaged in 24 sessions of play therapy when she was 17 years of age and a looked-after (foster) child. At the age of 18, she moved to the home of her mother's ex-boyfriend. He had been a positive male role model in her life and promised to support her in her quest for independent living. They moved to another city for employment, so that Irena was away from her previous support systems.

When Irena was 20, her worker contacted the therapist to request a follow-up session, as she had recently reconnected with Irena. Few details were provided except to share that Irena had been the victim of sex trafficking.

Irena arrived for her session and asked if she could go directly to the sandtray room, as she didn't want to talk. She used 30 minutes of the session to build a divided world. In one half of the world, a girl was placed in a lying position on a bed. Ariel (the Little Mermaid) was in another area of the tray, swimming and with shells near her, and, at the other end of the tray, there were a few windows, a police officer holding a radio and a filling station with an ambulance nearby.

Fifteen minutes before the session ended, Irena broke silence and asked the therapist if she knew the story. She then proceeded to tell the story of a young woman who was locked in a room where men would come in and hurt her. She would imagine herself to be a mermaid who could swim away without being violated. One day, the window in her room was unlocked, and her captor was watching television loudly in the next room. Though snow was on the ground and she only had underwear on, she was able to jump out of the window and run to the closest building, which was a filling station, where she used a phone to contact the police. An ambulance came, and they covered her with blankets, took her to the hospital, took care of her cold and cut feet and called her worker.

Irena described the second window as being the window of her future. Even with these experiences of hurt, Irena described the girl as being strong, with internal superpowers. She could imagine herself in peaceful places to overcome the incidents of abuse and overcome her embarrassment at being 'almost naked' to run, barefoot, for help in the snow.

We reviewed an earlier strategy, which was to journal three things daily that she was appreciative of in her life. This had proved to be very helpful for Irena as a teen in her development of relationships and resiliency factors. Irena shared that she had purchased a journal soon after being 'saved'. Irena talked about being happy about again living in her old community, near her foster parents and high-school friends. When asked about next steps, she said she didn't know, as she was just going to be happy for now feeling safe. She thanked the therapist for the opportunity to share her story and said if she needed another session she would call.

Her worker followed up a week later, thanking the therapist for her work and noting that Irena seemed more positive about her future. She also shared that Irena was more animated in her interactions with others. The worker noted that she was surprised so much was accomplished in one session.

Irena was able to move straight to narrating a coherent story of her experience using the miniature symbols, as the sandtray offered a safe and protected space. Initially, this was wordless to reflect her embodied experience and raw emotions (right hemisphere). This externalization may have facilitated Irena in adding language (left hemisphere) to facilitate understanding. The inclusion of a second window, into the future, may have facilitated processing, restoration of hope and the transformation of the implicit memories. Irena had previously established a meaningful relationship with the therapist, and that therapeutic intervention had helped to restructure the lower elements of the hierarchy of the brain, thus allowing Irena to move straight to therapeutic work that involved the limbic and cortical systems.

In this case the therapist was just present to hold the space and witness the story, which was full of symbolism of hope and survival. This sandtray was an example of resilience in the face of traumatic experiences.

## Conclusion

Contemporary neurobiological research has done much to inform creative and therapeutic interventions for those who work with children, adolescents, adults and families (e.g. Perry and Hambrick, 2008; Siegel, 2012; Schore, 2013). Neurosequential approaches take account of the hierarchical organization of the brain and the need for state regulation prior to cortical-oriented interventions. Storytelling and narrative are valuable tools for creative psychotherapy and are well suited to work with clients across the lifespan. They engage the higher-functioning areas of the brain, the limbic and cortical systems, through bottom–up interventions or top–down approaches. A social, interpersonal context is provided by the therapist's empathetic understanding and the therapeutic relationship.

## Key points

- Storytelling and narrative support the development of the limbic and cortical systems.
- Wordless storytelling precedes verbal storytelling.
- Regulation of emotions is supported by the acknowledgement and naming of feelings when a supportive adult narrates the child's experience and names their feelings.
- The higher-functioning cortical system manages the limbic system by piecing together a coherent narrative.
- Storytelling supports the integration of the brain by developing smooth connections between the right hemisphere, which is focused on the context of an experience and functions in a sensorial framework, and the left hemisphere, which is focused on the content of the experience and functions in a linear, logical manner.
- Choosing an intervention at this level assumes either that interventions have already targeted the lower brain regions or that the development of previous systems in the sequence had not been compromised.

## References

Bateman, A., Danby, S., and Howard, J. (2013a). Living in a broken world: How young children's well-being is supported through playing out their earthquake experiences. *International Journal of Play*, 2(3), 202–19.

Bateman, A., Danby, S., and Howard, J. (2013b). Everyday preschool talk about the Christchurch earthquakes. *Australian Journal of Communication*, 40(1), 103–22.

Bateman, A., Danby, S., and Howard, J. (2015). A review of the analysis of children's conversations about traumatic events. In M. O'Reilly and J. Nina Lester (eds) *The Palgrave Handbook of Child Mental Health*. Basingstoke, UK: Palgrave Macmillan.

Blake, Q. (1990). *All Join In*. London: Random House Children's Books.

Bolton, G. (1999). *The Therapeutic Potential of Creative Writing: Writing myself.* London: Jessica Kingsley.

Bruner, J.S., and Lucariello, J. (1989). Monologue as narrative recreation of the world. In K. Nelson (ed.) *Narratives from the Crib* (pp. 73–97). Cambridge, MA: Harvard University Press.

Damasio, A. (1999). *The Feeling of what Happened: The body and emotion in the making of consciousness*. San Diego, CA: Harcourt.

Eammons, R.A., and McCullough, M.E. (2003). Counting blessings versus burdens: An experimental investigation of gratitude and subjective well-being in daily life. *Journal of Personality & Social Psychology, 84*(2), 377–89.

Howard, J., and McInnes, K. (2012). The impact of children's perception of an activity as play rather than not play on emotional well-being. *Child Care, Health & Development, 39*(5), 737–42.

Howard, J., and McInnes, K. (2013). *The Essence of Play: A practice companion for professionals working with children and young people*. London: Routledge.

Kestly, T. (2015). Sandtray and storytelling in play therapy. In A. Stewart and D. Crenshaw (eds) *Play Therapy: A comprehensive guide to theory and practice*. New York: Guilford Press.

Mills, J., and Crowley, R. (1986). *Therapeutic Metaphors for Children and the Child Within*. New York: Brunner/Mazel.

Nicolopoulou, A. (2006). Interplay of play and narrative in children's development: Theoretical reflections and concrete examples. In A. Goncu and S. Gaskins (eds) *Play and Development: Evolutionary, sociocultural and functional perspectives*. Mahwah, NJ: Erlbaum.

Panksepp, J. (1998). *Affective Neuroscience: The foundations of human and animal emotions*. New York: Oxford University Press.

Pennebaker, J.W. (2000). Telling stories: The health benefits of narrative. *Literature and Medicine, 19*(1), 3–18.

Perry, B.D. (2006). Applying principles of neurodevelopment to clinical work with maltreated and traumatized children. A neurosequential model of therapeutics. In N. Boyd Webb (ed.) *Working with Traumatized Youth in Child Welfare* (pp. 27–52). New York: Guilford Press

Perry, B.D., and Hambrick, E. (2008). The neurosequential model of therapeutics. *Reclaiming Children & Youth, 17*(3), 38–43.

Perry, B.D., and Szalavitz, M. (2006). *The Boy Who Was Raised as a Dog*. New York: Basic Books.

Perry, B.D. (2001). The neuroarcheology of childhood treatment: The neurodevelopmental costs of adverse childhood events. In K. Franey, R. Geffner and R. Falconer (eds) *The Cost of Maltreatment: Who pays? We all do* (pp. 15–37). San Diego, CA: Family Violence and Sexual Assault Institute.

Schore, A. (2013). Joy and fun, gene, neurobiology and child brain development. [online video]. Available at: www.youtube.com/watch?v=Y0iocZu1mVg (accessed 27 May 2016).

Shore, R. (1997). *Rethinking the Brain: New insights into early development.* New York: Families and Work Institute.
Siegel, D. (2010). *Mindsight.* Oxford, UK: Oneworld.
Siegel, D. (2012). *The Developing Mind* (2nd edn). London: Guildford Press.
Siegel, D., and Bryson, T.P. (2011). *The Whole-Brain Child: 12 revolutionary strategies to nurture your child's developing mind.* New York: Delacorte Press.
Smith, C. (1997). Comparing traditional therapies with narrative approaches. In C. Smith and D. Nylund (eds) *Narrative Therapies with Children and Adolescents.* New York: Guilford Press.
Sunderland, M. (2006). *The Science of Parenting.* New York: DK Publishing.
Taylor de Faoite, A. (2011). *Narrative Play Therapy: Theory and practice.* London: Jessica Kingsley.
Trevarthen, C. (1995). The child's need to learn a culture. *Children and Society*, 9, 5–19.

Chapter 11

# A growing brain – a growing imagination

*Karen Stagnitti*

## Introduction

This chapter explores drama and imaginative play as expressed through pretend play as a lifespan activity. Research in brain development is beginning to identify the many regions in the limbic and cortex regions that are activated when children and adults engage in pretend-play scenarios. Although this research is still in the first decade of studies, already it has been found that neural activation through watching pretend-play scenarios is associated with brain regions linked to social and emotional understanding (theory of mind), narrative language and self-regulation. These findings provide evidence for the timing and use of activities that facilitate pretend-play ability within play therapies that are informed by the developmental neurosequential framework. In this chapter, examples of pretend-play activities are given for a child who was involved in sessions that used a Learn to Play therapy approach, an adolescent who was involved in a small group where group activities were informed by the Learn to Play approach, and an adult who was able to integrate emotional distress through an adult form of pretend play, improvisation. Play is powerful. It is powerful because social, emotional, narrative and sense of self can be integrated through play.

## Drama and imaginative play in psychotherapeutic practice

Drama and imaginative play involve imposing meaning on a situation and creating a scene or a series of scenes. In her work, Sue Jennings uses the term 'dramatic play' for the developmental progression of the child from birth to 7 years. She stated that, 'dramatic development of children . . . is the basis of a child being able to enter the world of imagination and symbolism' (Jennings, 2014: 82). Symbolism, pretence and social interaction are involved in drama and imaginative play, and these abilities require engagement of the limbic and cortical systems in the brain. As both drama and imaginative play involve symbols and pretence, pretend play will be the focus of this chapter, including how it changes and develops from childhood to adolescence to adulthood. Underpinning this discussion is the recognition that true play is dynamic and fun (Eberle, 2014; Gaskill and Perry, 2014). True play is pleasure, surprise, anticipation, understanding, strength and poise (Eberle, 2014). It is not obsession, compulsion, terror, indifference and heedlessness (Eberle, 2014). There is joy when we are truly playing. Sunderland (2007) argues that true play is good brain chemistry, as there is a release of a symphony of 'feel good' hormones such as opioids, oxytocin and dopamine when we are engaged in physically interactive play. Children, adolescents or adults who find no pleasure in age-appropriate pretend play or physically interactive play are argued to be at risk of poorer well-being than those who enjoy such activities (Miller and Almon, 2009; Gray, 2011; Capps, 2012; Eberle, 2014).

Pretend play (also called dramatic play, imaginative play, representational play, make-believe play, fantasy play) develops in the second year of life and can be observed in the child imitating others in their social context (also see Jennings, 2014). For example, a 12-month-old who is holding an empty cup and pretending to have a drink is showing a play script that reflects their daily life, while imposing meaning that the empty cup has liquid in it that you can drink. By 2 years of age, a child can order their play actions sequentially: for example, putting blocks in a truck and pushing it or feeding a teddy and then putting the teddy to bed (Stagnitti, 2009). Children tell stories about themselves (Stagnitti and Jellie, 2006), and their emerging self-representations are tied to behaviours (for example, 'I am strong. I can lift the truck') as they overestimate their abilities (Harter, 2012). In these early years, significant adults help a child to understand their autobiographical narrative (Harter, 2012), with self-recognition related to autobiographical memories (Lewis and Carmody, 2008). Measures of self-representation in small children are recognition of self in a mirror, usage of personal pronouns and pretend play (Lewis and Carmody, 2008). These autobiographical memories can be observed in a child's pretend play, as play in these early years reflects the child's daily life story. Perry (2009) notes the importance of repetition, and certainly repetition can be observed in young children's pretend play scripts: for example, having lots of cups of tea at a tea party or repeated actions of putting in blocks and pushing the truck, taking blocks out and putting blocks in. By 3 years, a child's range of play scenarios expands, as they weave in fictional characters and parts of previously known story plots in their play. Children play for longer and begin to pre-plan their play by thinking about what to play before they begin (Stagnitti, 1998). By this age, Rakoczy (2008a, 2008b) argues, children understand that they are playing intentionally with others, and that play reflects implicit rules that reflect the conventions of their social and cultural environments (see also Nicolopoulou *et al.*, 2010). The emergence of pretend play, together with interactions with others in social play, involves a child's understanding and 'reading' of social situations, which was coined 'theory of mind', a term used to explain a child's understanding of the mental states of others as well as their own (Hughes and Leekam, 2004; Lewis and Carmody, 2008). Increasing ability in joint social pretend play reflects the implicit rules reflecting conventions within the child's cultural context, with children showing understanding of mental states of others through their pretend play (Rakoczy, 2008a, 2008b; Stagnitti, 2015). Although a link between theory of mind and pretend play has been demonstrated, evidence of a causal link between social pretend play and theory of mind has still not been established (Dore *et al.*, 2015). By preschool, children can play out a story script over 2–3 days to 2–3 weeks, embed problems in the play and become a character in the play while engaging with several peers (Stagnitti, 1998; Whittington and Floyd, 2009). Through conversation and talking about the play as they play (called 'metaplay'; see Pellegrini and Galda, 1993), children create joint shared meanings in their pretend play, and these joint meanings in social play require the child to think logically to extend on the ideas of others, introduce a new idea or prop and use verbal and nonverbal communication with peers about whether they accept or reject a peer's idea (Whittington and Floyd, 2009). Thinking logically and extending on the ideas of others produce a play narrative, and, when that narrative includes characters, the child is demonstrating their understanding that individuals have differing beliefs and viewpoints (Stagnitti, 2015). Narrative involves social–perceptual theory of mind, because producing a narrative involves relating a sequentially organized set of events in time and space, with embedded problems seen from different perspectives and emotional states of the characters involved (Stirling *et al.*, 2014; Stagnitti, 2015). During these early years of developing pretend play, children with high self-esteem show confidence, curiosity, initiative and independence in their play (Harter, 2012). Preschool children with higher levels of complexity in their play are more likely to be socially competent with peers (McAloney and Stagnitti, 2009) and have been found to have more complex language and narrative skills 4 years later, when they were in early primary school (Stagnitti and Lewis, 2015). The impact of pretend play on a child's development was critiqued by Lillard, Lerner *et al.* (2013) to determine whether pretend play was crucial (that is, causal to development), equifinal (that is, pretend play is one possible route impacting some aspects of development) or an epiphenomenon (that is, occurs alongside development but of itself makes no contribution). They concluded that pretend play was: possibly crucial to language, narrative and emotion regulation; equifinal to reasoning and possibly equifinal to theory of mind, social skills, language and narrative; and epiphenomenal possibly to creativity, intelligence, reasoning, conservation, theory of mind, social skills and language. Lillard, Lerner *et al.* (2013) and Lillard, Hopkins *et al.* (2013) noted methodological issues in the vast majority of the studies that included confusion in the definition and measurement of pretend play, bias of researchers, and research design. They put forward valuable suggestions for future research. Although the paper is an important paper, it must be noted that the literature critiqued was not exhaustive: for example, research on creativity by Sandra Russ or evidence on play therapy by Dee Ray or Sue Bratton (for example, see Ray *et al.*, 2001) were not referred to.

In middle childhood, children develop the ability to play one game over longer time periods and stop games and revisit them later (Bergen and Fromberg, 2009; Kuhaneck *et al.*, 2010). From 5 to 7 years, a child's autobiographical narrative begins to be crafted within their cultural norms, and the child takes an increasing role in constructing their own autobiographical narrative (Harter, 2012). Self-descriptive terms can reflect labels modelled by others, however; children don't yet 'own' these views of the self by others (Harter, 2012). Theory of mind continues to develop, with children now understanding that others have different viewpoints, motives and beliefs, and can cover true emotions (Hughes and Leekam, 2004; Harter, 2012). Middle childhood may also be a time where some children feel pressure from parents, older siblings and peers to 'grow up' (Manning, 2006), with pretending seen as a younger child's domain. However, it has been found that, through play, children are able to practise communication, negotiation, organization and conflict-resolution skills while playing with their peers (Bergen and Fromberg, 2009). When engaged in dramatic role-playing, children learn to control their thought processes and practise coping strategies for use in real-life situations (Singer, 2006). Children who access and use affective themes in their pretend play have a better understanding of their own and others' emotions (Seja and Russ, 1999), and children who engage in pretend play have better divergent thinking and problem-solving skills (Russ et al., 1999).

Gaskill and Perry (2014) rightly argue that play changes form as children develop. Pretend play changes form from middle childhood to adolescence. Daydreaming, a form of creative thinking and pretending, was found to occur during daily life in 38 per cent of a student sample with a mean age of 18.7 years (Smith and Lillard, 2012). Hence, pretending flips from playing on the floor with toys to being a mental process that informs social communication. Early adolescence brings a greater awareness of false-self behaviour, such as concealing true thoughts and feelings and the detection of hypocrisy in others more than themselves (Harter, 2012). There is an increased critical evaluation of others and sensitivity to others' comments (Harter, 2012). Thus, increasing complexity in theory of mind and understanding others is heightened in early adolescence. Peer relationships are particularly salient in an adolescent's life (Peake et al., 2013), and, if adolescents do not have the ability to socially interact, they are at risk of being socially isolated (Goldingay et al., 2015). Appropriate recognition of emotions in others, self-regulation, the ability to negotiate and flexible thinking are now important abilities for the adolescent so that they can enter and be part of social situations with their peer group (Goldingay et al., 2015). Goldingay et al. (2015) found that adolescents with social difficulties lacked fundamental complex pretend play ability, as they showed difficulties in formulating fictional scenarios with extended narratives that included characters and symbols.

Göncü and Perone (2005) have argued that pretend play is a lifelong activity, with the example of improvisation as a form of age-appropriate adult pretend play. In their paper, they argued that the underlying ability of pretend play contributed to emotional regulation in adulthood. Whitehead et al. (2009) investigated areas of the brain that were activated when adults were engaged in watching a pretend play activity (for example, using a tennis racquet as a guitar). They found that the limbic and cortical areas of an adult's brain were activated, including areas associated with theory of mind, imagining situations and understanding emotional gestures (medial prefrontal cortex, posterior superior temporal sulcus and temporal poles) and areas associated with narrative (such as the ventrolateral prefrontal, orbitomedial prefrontal areas, inferior parietal and dorsolateral frontal lobe and posterior cingulate; Whitehead *et al.*, 2009).

To summarize, theory of mind and pretend play have been argued to be interlinked (Baron-Cohen, 1996; Hughes and Leekam, 2004), although a causal link has not yet been established (Dore *et al.*, 2015). Pretend play development in childhood is linked to narrative, language, social competence and emotion regulation – skills needed throughout life – with Lillard, Lerner *et al.* (2013) concluding that it may be possible that pretend play is crucial or equifinal to the first three and possibly crucial to emotion regulation. However, much more rigorous research is required. The next section will consider pretend play in conjunction with the neurosequential model.

## Pretend play and neurosequential development

The neurosequential development of the brain is hierarchical, with the organization of the brain moving from the brainstem (least complex) to the cortex (most complex; Perry, 2009). Each of the four main regions of the brain (brainstem, diencephalon, limbic system and cortex) develops and becomes fully functional during different periods of a person's development (Perry, 2009). The least complex areas of the brain develop first and influence the continued development of more complex areas (Perry, 2009). The approach of the neurosequential model of therapeutics (Perry and Hambrick, 2008; Perry, 2009), when working with children and adolescents who have experienced trauma and developmental difficulties, is to begin work with the lowest functioning regions of the brain and work up to more complex areas of the brain as improvements are seen. According to the neurosequential model, play at the limbic and cortical level encourages abstract thought and storytelling, drama and theatre (Perry, 2006). Pretend play is about imposing meaning and storytelling. Pretend play begins to develop from approximately 12 to 18 months of age, when the least complex areas of the brain are more influential than the cortical regions (Perry, 2009), and continues into adolescence and adulthood, when the cortex is fully functional (Perry, 2009; Smith *et al.*, 2013). As the cortex takes years before it is fully organized and functional (Perry, 2009), pretend play takes years before it becomes highly complex. Complex pretend play incorporates the ability to sequentially and logically think through self-initiated narratives in play with embedded problems that are resolved with reference to temporal sequences, character beliefs and motivations, role-play, use of symbols and the ability to decentre from self (Stagnitti, 2015). The activity of pretend play over time changes from playing on the floor with toys to age-appropriate activity forms, such as drama, school musicals, improvisation and the ability to follow complex emotional and social behaviours in interactions of others.

Over the past decade or so, the activity that occurs in the brain when people are engaged in pretend play has been investigated. Findings have confirmed that pretend-play engagement is associated with neural activation in the limbic and cortical regions of the brain (Whitehead *et al.*, 2009), and this is consistent with knowledge of neurosequential development (Perry and Hambrick, 2008; Perry, 2009). In a study exploring self-representation and brain development in children aged 15–30 months, the degree of brain maturation in the left temporo-parietal junction (the temporal lobes are associated with the limbic system and cortex structures) was related to the emergence of a child's self-representation (Lewis and Carmody, 2008). Three other measures of self-representation (recognition of self in the mirror, spontaneous pretend play and use of personal pronouns) were also associated with maturation in this area of the brain (Lewis and Carmody, 2008).

The association between pretend play and theory of mind has been investigated, with the measure of theory of mind being the false-belief task (Hughes and Leekam, 2004). The false-belief task is when an individual (such as yourself) understands the views of all the characters in a story and can accurately predict the actions of a character in the story who does not know the truth. Kuhn-Popp *et al.* (2013) argued that pretend play and false belief both require mental processes in the higher levels of the brain. In Kuhn-Popp *et al.*'s study, children aged 6 and 8 years were presented with a pretend-play scenario and a false-belief scenario in cartoon form. In children aged 6–8 years, frontal activity in the brain (cortical area) was found during both pretend-play reasoning and false-belief reasoning. In children, pretend-play actions were related to intention (Kuhn-Popp *et al.*, 2013). For the false-belief scenario, Kuhn-Popp *et al.* (2013) argued that false belief requires metarepresentation (the representation of the representational relation towards truth). Developmentally, Kuhn-Popp *et al.*'s study found that, in children, neural activity in the cortex showed diffuse activity with less-localized frontal activity, and they argued this was related to substantial structural changes and ongoing neural specialization, with ongoing development in the cortex. The findings seem to substantiate accounts by Rakoczy (2008a, 2008b), who argued children have intention in their reasoning in pretend play (Kuhn-Popp *et al.*, 2013).

In a study with adults, Whitehead *et al.* (2009) found that, when adults watched a pretend-play scenario (for example, a tennis racquet used as a guitar), the limbic and cortical regions of the brain associated with theory of mind and narrative were activated. A considerable overlap between studies of narrative and studies of theory of mind may be due to many theory-of-mind studies using narrative stimuli, as narrative requires emotional and social understanding of a character's intentions and scenarios (Whitehead *et al.*, 2009). From their study, Whitehead *et al.* (2009) put forward that pretend play 'is a form of communicative narrative' (p. 369) associated with the ability to imagine a scenario. Smith *et al.* (2013) largely confirmed Whitehead *et al.*'s findings (2009), even though there were differences in methodology. Smith *et al.* (2013) found that, when adult participants viewed videos of an actor in a pretend-play scenario carrying out an action with no object (the imaginative scenario) and an action using an object with no physical similarity to the intended object (such as using a spoon as a saw), the inferior frontal gyrus was activated, which is implicated in theory-of-mind processes. The middle frontal gyrus, also implicated in theory of mind, was activated in imaginary pretence. The fusiform gyrus, which is involved in a wide range of sociocognitive scenarios, and the precuneus (also found to activate when participants consider beliefs, desires and intentions of others), inferior parietal lobule, fusiform and the superior parietal lobule were all activated when people viewed videos of people engaged in various forms of pretend play acting.

Hence, studies with children and adults have confirmed that there is limbic–cortical activation when participants are engaged in watching and thinking about pretend-play scenarios, and this activation is associated with theory of mind (social cognition), narrative (language) and self-regulation. Findings in these studies are consistent with neurosequential development, where more complex cortical functions take longer to mature. This parallels the development of pretend play, which begins in the second year of life and continues through to adulthood.

Figure 11.1 is a schematic representation of the developmental progression of pretend play as it develops from early play abilities, where the child's play is primarily physical and sensory play, through to pretend play in childhood, which develops further and changes form in adolescence and adulthood. The next section of this chapter describes three case studies with activities related to pretend play.

## Drama and imaginative play practice with a child: A case study

Marley, a male child aged 8 years, was referred by a local community-based service for Learn to Play therapy (Stagnitti, 1998), because his pretend-play ability was delayed by 5 years. The Learn to Play therapy approach is a child-centred approach that was influenced by Axline's non-directive play therapy (Axline, 1947). The child is accepted unconditionally; a warm relationship is built with the child; the child's capacity to develop is respected; there is a permissive atmosphere to therapy, as the child is free to self-initiate; and the therapist responds to the child's lead (Stagnitti, 1998, 2009, 2014). The Learn to Play therapy approach facilitates the development of a child's ability to self-initiate pretend play through skills such as: play scripts, sequences of play actions, object substitution, social interaction, role-play and character play (Stagnitti, 1998).

Marley presented as a well-looked-after child who lived with his grandparents and older brother. His parents had been killed in a car accident when he was 3 years old. He found it difficult to concentrate at school and was behind in his learning. In his play, he found it difficult to maintain a long sequence of actions, which resulted in his play moving constantly from one idea to another with little connection. He also had difficulty with symbols in play (object substitution) and was quite literal in his use of objects (for example, the blocks were used to build a tower, the box was to put other objects in it). Being aware that this child had

## 192  Karen Stagnitti

**Pretend play**
Increasing complexity from 12-18 months to late childhood

**Representational thought evidenced by:** object substitution (symbols in play), referring to absent objects, attribution of properties. Reference to something or someone outside of self (decentration), social pretend play, role play with emersion of characters in the play. Logical sequential thought, narrative, problem solving (divergent and convergent thinking), flexibility and adaptability in thinking, metacognition, 'metaplay' (talking about the play as you play)

**In adolescence and adulthood:** understanding of social rules, social perceptiveness, perception of context – emotional and social, formulation of arguments

**Early play**
Predominates in first 2 years

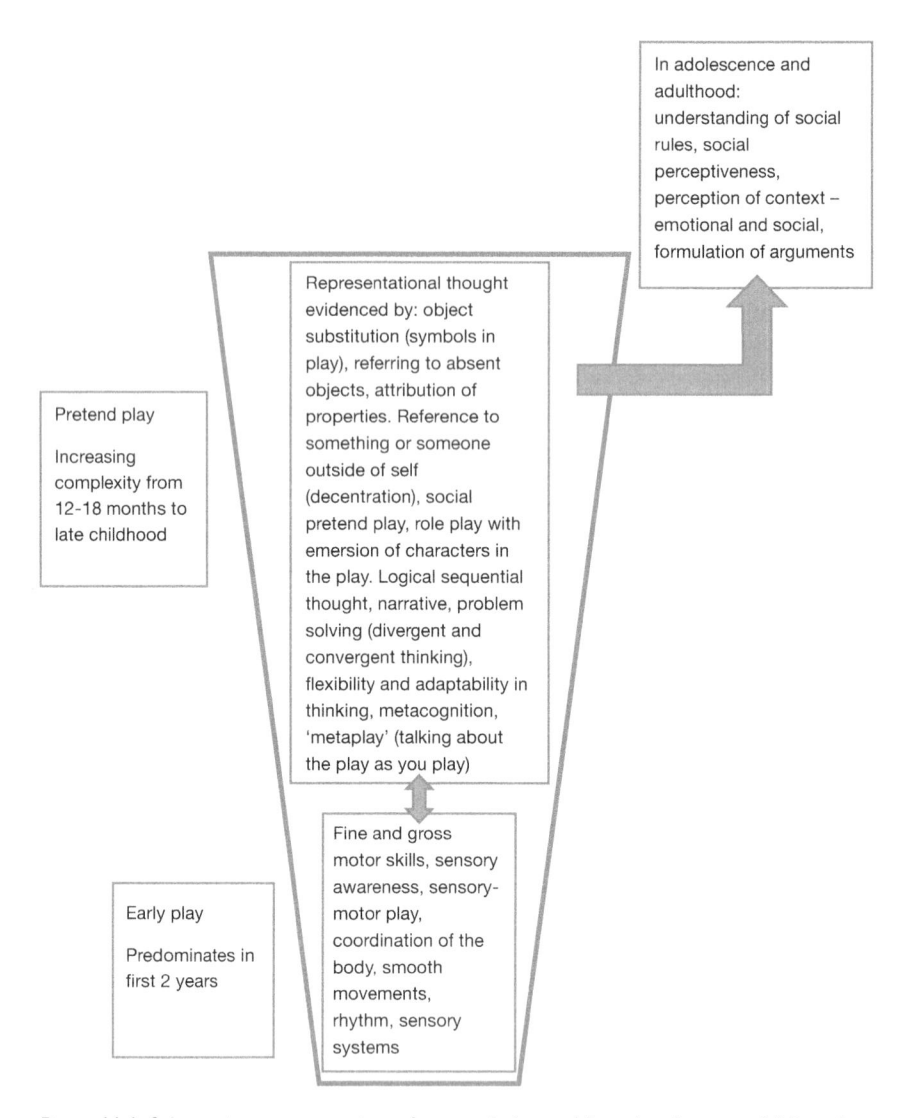

Fine and gross motor skills, sensory awareness, sensory-motor play, coordination of the body, smooth movements, rhythm, sensory systems

*Figure 11.1* Schematic representation of pretend play and how it relates to childhood, adolescents and adults

experienced a traumatic event (the death of his parents at a young age) and that his play ability could be a combination of a reaction to this trauma as well as possibly his own developmental difficulties, the activity planed for Marley began with a Learn to Play therapy approach.

Therapy began on the level of Marley's pretend-play ability. The therapist modelled play scripts that were familiar to Marley and that involved only four or five play actions in a sequence. There was minimal use of object substitution to begin with, and the play scenarios reflected domestic and life scripts that allowed for repetition with variation. Examples of the play activities were: taking the teddies fishing and catching, cooking and eating the fish; creating a zoo and having buses of people (small character dolls) going on the bus to see the animals; cooking dinner with teddy bear; and people riding on a train and then going shopping. These pretend-play scripts were modelled by the therapist using only the play props necessary for the play scene (so as not to overwhelm Marley), responding to Marley by either extending or retracting the number of play actions in a sequence (hence, creating either more or less complex play scenes) and gradually introducing symbols in play (such as a box for the train). When working with Marley, the therapist was constantly responding to him, ensuring there was a safe environment and taking the play to earlier play forms (involving lower brain regions), such as sensory play, if Marley showed signs of being overwhelmed (such as disengaging from the play, piling the toys up in front of him on the floor or verbalizing his wish to finish playing). After 3 months, Marley was beginning to show increased ability in self-initiation of pretend-play action sequences and he was adding to the play and extending the play without prompting or modelling from the therapist. It was then, when Marley's pretend play was becoming more complex, that he began to use pretend play scenarios that reflected underlying emotional states, such as feelings of abandonment, dying, never having enough, anger and frustration. The activity plan then moved to non-directive play sessions, where Marley could choose any toys from any of the shelves and cupboards in the room, and the therapist took a physically more passive role, while being verbally responsive using tracking and empathetic reflection. Over time, Marley's play themes reflected trust, safety, protection, mastery and a sense of completion. The development of a child's ability to engage in pretend play that was at the pace of the child, where the child felt safe, not only enabled the child to increase his complex play skills, which has implications for increased social competence with peers and increased narrative language and self-regulation, but also allowed Marley to work through his emotional trauma from the death of his parents 5 years earlier.

## Drama and imaginative play practice with an adolescent: A case study

Susan was a 14-year-old teen who had been referred by her school welfare officer because she had great difficulties with social interaction with peers. She could be impulsive and volatile and become overwhelmed when there were several events occurring at the same time (such as people near her talking, someone wanting her to look at a picture on their phone and the teacher demanding attention from the group). Susan had four siblings, all older, and her parents worked full time. The family were a loving family; however, they were a busy family with little time to spend with their children. The Learn to Play therapy approach for adolescents is based on the assumption that adolescents who experience social difficulties and lack flexibility with peers and/or are literal in their thinking have not developed pretend play to the level of complexity that was required before the onset of puberty. High levels of complex play involve the ability to use symbols in play that do not necessarily reflect the physical properties of the intended object (for example, a chair could be a rocket); the ability to understand the logical sequence of play actions that results in a narrative with embedded problems and resolutions that may extend over several weeks; and the ability to use language to describe a scene, set the context of the play and explain the roles, motivations and beliefs of characters within the play, while keeping track of the mental states of several people simultaneously. These abilities also bring with them flexibility in thought, practice in negotiation with peers and the ability to think forward and plan ahead what will happen next. The Animated Movie Test, developed by Karen Stagnitti (and undergoing refinement at the time of writing), is a test of pretend play in an age-appropriate form for young people aged from 12 to 18 years. The young person is presented with seven prop boxes and instructed that they are the director of an animated movie and the props are their movie props. They have 15 minutes to set up the movie and 15 minutes to produce the movie. It has been found that young people with social difficulties can set up the movie but have great difficulty producing the movie narrative (Goldingay *et al.*, 2015). Susan reflected this, as her movie was a literal telling of the props on the table, with some functional relationships between the props. For example, the horse and dog jumped about, the man came to the horse and patted the horse, the man gave the horse some food, the dog barked, and the horse ate the food.

Susan began the activities with a small group of five other adolescents aged 13–15 years. As adolescence is a time where peer groups and peer pressure are prominent (Peake *et al.*, 2013), a Learn to Play approach for adolescents involves work in small groups (see Goldingay *et al.*, 2015). The group was conducted at Susan's school for 1 hour once a week during school term. Learn to Play for adolescents is an 8-week programme where a small group of adolescents work towards producing a movie. To do this, they are required to engage with abilities that underpin pretend play, such as development of characters, the narrative sequence and the use of symbols in the movie, while working together as a group to negotiate the narrative. The weekly group structure is designed to be predictable and create a safe space for the group. A warm-up activity begins the group, followed by staged activities each week that scaffold the group to create a movie together. These warm-up activities focus on age-appropriate development of object substitution (use of symbols), theory-of-mind scenarios using popular figurines (such as characters from popular movies or TV series) or autobiographical activities such as bringing an object that reflects who they are. The techniques used by facilitators are scaffolding and modelling, repetition with variation (similar activities over 2 or 3 weeks that expand on a similar ability or topic) and ensuring the complexity of the tasks are at the level of the group. To achieve a group production of a short movie, the adolescents work in pairs to discuss possible movie story topics, character development and scenes. The pairs of adolescents then join together to discuss their ideas, and further negotiation is facilitated to agree on an overarching narrative, which could include ideas from all the pairs. Being underpinned by neurosequential development, activities that reflected less complex neural regions (brainstem and midbrain) are also included at appropriate times if the activities pitched at the cortical level begin to overwhelm the group. At these times, activities such as drumming and rhythm are used to settle the group and provide a sense of calm and safety. Stress balls are also used by the young people when sitting and listening.

Initially, Susan was chatty in the group, but, when asked a direct question, she would blush and struggled to speak. In the warm-up activity where alternative uses for a cloth were discussed, Susan came up with two uses. By the third session, the group facilitators introduced and modelled to the group the use of a story board. The story board included both pictures and text, so that the group could visualize a narrative structure and how to develop a movie plot. Susan worked with one other group member to come up with a story. The facilitators then explained a story needs characters; in this case, characters were made out of soft clay. Susan enjoyed playing with the soft clay while listening to a warm-up activity where a story that required theory of mind was being told. At the end of this group, Susan had left her soft clay in pieces. Susan needed support to construct her character and, by the fourth week, she began working with the soft clay to develop her movie character. By the fourth week, warm-up activities included theory-of-mind scenarios using figurines. Susan had difficulty understanding the character's false belief in the scenario, and it was not until three further theory-of-mind scenarios had been presented to the group that she began to grasp the concept. By the fifth week, the group watched a 1-minute clip of a movie that had no sound. Susan could articulate the feelings of the characters, but had difficulty thinking of possible events that might have led to the feelings of the character. By week six, Susan had made her character for the movie and was able to describe different physical attributes, but struggled to articulate motives or beliefs. As a group, they needed scaffolding to decide on a group story structure with beginning, problem in the middle and then the resolution to the problem. Susan appeared to get lost in the group and used her stress ball throughout the group session. The facilitators scaffolded more structure and guided each group member in choosing a role to play in the movie. For example, there was the artistic director, the set designer, the overall director, the narrator, the main script writer. Susan opted to be the set designer. As they settled into roles, and the movie narrative began to develop, Susan could carry out her role as set designer by drawing the backdrops to the movie scenes. There were five movie scenes, and, by the end of week seven, all five scenes were prepared, the narrative was laid out on the story board, the characters were ready, and the script included a beginning, a problem and a resolution. By week eight, the group was enthusiastic to film their movie. As Susan had a set role, she was comfortable staying with her allocated role and, by the end of the group, was smiling and enjoying the playful interaction. The school requested that the group run for the rest of the school year, and Susan was agreeable to keep attending. The facilitators noted that she was becoming more self-confident and was beginning to be more aware of the intent of the social interactions in the group.

## Drama and imaginative play practice with an adult: A case study

Play is necessary throughout life, and, as an age-appropriate adult activity, pretend play takes the form of painting, poetry, dance, theatre, cinema, performance and festive activities (Göncü and Perone, 2005). Göncü and Perone also consider improvisation an example of adult pretend play. The parallels between pretend play and improvisation are that they both have symbolic activity and free-flowing spontaneous engagement. They are both social in nature, where negotiation, development of characters, narrative and turn-taking occur, and emotional engagement is required (Göncü and Perone, 2005). In this case scenario, pretend play, in the form of improvisation, was used to help Paul make sense of his experiences of a recent divorce, where he was left bereft, with a sense of helplessness. He was in his 30s and had been married for 10 years. There were no children, but his vision of his future had included children. He was in a steady job and had come from a childhood where there was a stable home background. Both his parents had died from a chronic disease when he was in his late 20s. His wife leaving him had come as a shock. He had not picked up any emotional incongruences between himself and his wife. She had left him for someone else.

A friend had become concerned about Paul's mental health and had encouraged him to join him in a social group once a week, where improvisation was the main form of interaction, and group members were the audience. Paul had not heard of improvisation and was reticent to join; however, when his friend came to pick him up, Paul felt he should just go, because it would take too much energy to resist. In Göncü and Perone's words, adult improvation is 'a social pretend activity involving negotiation and working through of experiences among the actors' (2005: 143). Paul was quiet and sat on the side for the first session. He watched and found himself immersed in the social interactions, playfulness and safety of the group. Emotionally, he found he had transcended his situation and found a sense of relief at having left his current situation for the moment. Unexpectedly, even to himself, Paul agreed to attend the following week. By his third week of attendance, he began to join in, negotiating on the plot and character he would role-play. Week after week he immersed himself in different roles with different emotions and imagining different scenarios, separate to his life situation. He found himself smiling and realized he hadn't smiled for a long time. The involvement in improvisation gave him a safe environment to play out different feelings within a contained space, and he felt held by the group to be able to show his anger, despair, sadness and helplessness. Through this, his affect regulation became more stable, and he was able to concentrate and be more productive at work.

## Conclusion

Drama and imaginative play were captured by the term pretend play in this chapter. Pretend play is cognitive play activity that is neurologically associated with self-regulation, narrative and theory-of-mind understanding. Studies have confirmed that, when children and adults are engaged in pretend-play activity, neural activation occurs in the limbic and cortical regions of the brain, with children showing less-localized activity than adults owing to their developing brain. More complex regions of the brain take years to become fully functional, and pretend play reflects this complexity, being a lifespan activity from childhood to adulthood. The knowledge of pretend-play development, together with an understanding of how it links to theory of mind, narrative and self-regulation, can inform therapists when they are choosing developmentally appropriate activities. When these activities are targeted at the correct level of complexity, therapy reflects a neurosequential framework to facilitate social and emotional development throughout the lifespan.

## Key points

- Pretend play is a lifespan activity.
- Pretend play incorporates drama and imaginative play, which are neurologically associated with theory of mind (hence, social and emotional understanding), self-regulation and narrative.
- Activities for pretend play can begin at a 12–18-month level and increase in complexity as the individual develops their abilities.
- Activities in pretend play can be adjusted for age-appropriate activities in adolescence and adulthood.
- Therapists working at higher brain levels with children and adolescents in drama and imaginative-play activities can also introduce activities at lower brain levels when the drama and imaginative-play activities become too challenging.

## References

Axline, V. (1947). *Play Therapy*. New York: Ballantine Books.
Baron-Cohen, S. (1996). *Mindblindness: An essay on autism and theory of mind*. London: MIT Press.
Bergen, D., and Fromberg, D. (2009). Play and social interaction in middle childhood. *Phi Delta Kappan*, 90, 426–30.
Capps, D. (2012). Child's play: The creativity of older adults. *Journal of Religion & Health*, 51, 630–50.
Dore, R.A., Smith, E.D., and Lillard, A.S. (2015). How is theory of mind useful? Perhaps to enable social pretend play. *Frontiers in Psychology*, 6, 1–4.
Eberle, S.G. (2014). Elements of play. Toward a philosophy and definition of play. *Journal of Play*, 6(2), 214–33.

Gaskill, R., and Perry, B.D. (2014). The neurobiological power of play: Using the neurosequential model of therapeutics to guide play in the healing process. In C. Malchiodi and D. A Crenshaw (eds) *Play and Creative Arts Therapy for Attachment Trauma* (pp. 178–94). New York: Guilford Press.

Goldingay, S., Stagnitti, K., Sheppard, L., McGillivray, J., McLean, B., and Pepin, G. (2015). An intervention to improve social participation for adolescents with autism spectrum disorder: Pilot study. *Developmental Neurorehabilitation*, *18*(2), 122–30.

Göncü, A., and Perone, A. (2005). Pretend play as a lifespan activity. *Topoi*, *24*(2), 137–47.

Gray, P. (2011). The decline of play and rise of psychopathology in children and adolescents. *American Journal of Play*, *3*, 443–63.

Harter, S. (2012). *The Construction of the Self. Developmental and sociocultural foundations*. New York: Guilford Press.

Hughes, C., and Leekam, S. (2004). What are the links between theory of mind and social links? Review, reflections and new directions for studies of typical and atypical development. *Social Development*, *13*, 590–691.

Jennings, S. (2014). Applying an Embodiment–Projection–Role framework in groupwork with children. In E. Prendiville and J. Howard (eds) *Play Therapy Today. Contemporary practice with individuals, groups and carers* (pp. 79–96). London: Routledge.

Kuhaneck, H., Spitzer, S., and Miller, E. (2010). *Activity analysis, creativity, and playfulness in pediatric occupational therapy: Making play just right*. Sudbury, MA: Jones & Bartlett.

Kuhn-Popp, N., Sodian, B., Sommer, M. Dohnel, K., and Meinhardt, J. (2013). Same or different? ERP correlates of pretense and false belief reasoning in children. *Neuroscience*, *248*, 488–98.

Lewis, M., and Carmody, D. (2008). Self-representation and brain development. *Developmental Psychology*, *4*(5), 1329–34.

Lillard, A., Hopkins, E., Dore, R., Palmquist, C., Lerner, M., and Smith, E. (2013). Concepts and theories, methods and reasons: Why do the children (pretend) play? Reply to Weisberg, Hirsh-Pasek, and Golinkoff (2013); Bergen (2013); and Walker and Gopnik (2013). *Psychological Bulletin*, *139*(1), 49–52.

Lillard, A., Lerner, M., Hopkins, E., Dore, R., Smith, E., and Palmquist, C. (2013). The impact of pretend play on children's development: A review of the evidence. *Psychological Bulletin*, *139*(1), 1–34.

McAloney, K., and Stagnitti, K. (2009). Pretend play and social play: The concurrent validity of the child-initiated pretend play assessment. *International Journal of Play Therapy*, *18*(2), 99–113.

Manning, M.L. (2006). Play development from ages eight to twelve. In D.P. Fromberg and D. Bergen (eds) *Play from Birth to Twelve: Contexts, perspectives and meanings* (2nd edn, pp. 21–30). New York: Routledge.

Miller, E., and Almon, J. (2009). *Crisis in the Kindergarten. Why children need to play in school*. College Park, MD: Alliance for Childhood.

Nicolopoulou, N., Barbosa de Sá, A., Ilgaz, H., and Brockmeyer, C. (2010). Using the transformative power of play to educate hearts and minds: From Vygotsky to Vivian Paley and beyond. *Mind, Culture & Activity*, *17*(1), 42–58.

Peake, S, Dishion, T, Stormshak, E., and Moore, W. (2013). Risk-taking and social exclusion in adolescence: Neural mechanisms underlying peer influences on decision-making. *NeuroImage*, *82*, 23–34.

Pellegrini, A., and Galda, L. (1993). Ten years after: A re-examination of symbolic play and literacy research. *Reading Research Quarterly*, *28*, 163–75.

Perry, B.D. (2006). The neurosequential model of therapeutics: Applying principles of neuroscience to clinical work with traumatized and maltreated children. In N.B. Webb (ed.) *Working with Traumatized Youth in Child Welfare* (pp. 27–52). New York: Guilford Press.

Perry, B.D. (2009). Examining child maltreatment through a neurodevelopmental lens: Clinical applications of the neurosequential model of therapeutics. *Journal of Loss & Trauma*, *14*, 240–55.

Perry, B.D., and Hambrick, E. (2008). The neurosequential model of therapeutics. *Reclaiming Children & Youth*, *17*(3), 38–43.

Rakoczy, H. (2008a). Pretense as individual and collective intentionality. *Mind & Language*, *23*(5), 499–517.

Rakoczy, H. (2008b). Taking fiction seriously: Young children understand the normative structure of joint pretence games. *Developmental Psychology*, *44*, 1195–201.

Ray, D., Bratton, S., Rhine, T., and Jones, L. (2001). The effectiveness of play therapy: Responding to the critics. *International Journal of Play Therapy*, *10*(1), 85–108.

Russ, S.W., Robins, A.L., and Christiano, B.A. (1999). Pretend play: A longitudinal predication of creativity and affect in fantasy in children. *Creativity Research Journal*, *12*(2), 129–39.

Seja, A.L., and Russ, S.W. (1999). Children's fantasy play and emotional understanding. *Journal of Clinical Child Psychology*, *28*(2), 269–77.

Singer, J.L. (2006). Epilogue: Learning to play and learning through play. In D.G. Singer, R. Golinkoff and K. Hirsh-Pasek (eds) *Play = Learning: How play motivates and enhances children's cognitive and social-emotional growth* (pp. 251–62). New York: Oxford University Press.

Smith, E.D., Englander, Z.A., Lillard, A.S., and Morris, J.P. (2013). Cortical mechanisms of pretense observation. *Social Neuroscience*, *8*(4), 356–68.

Smith, E.D., and Lillard, A.S. (2012). Play on: Retrospective reports of the persistence of pretend play into middle childhood. *Journal of Cognition & Development*, *13*(4), 524–49.

Stagnitti, K. (1998). *Learn to Play: A practical program to develop a child's imaginative play*. Melbourne, VIC: Co-ordinates Publications.

Stagnitti, K. (2009). Play intervention: The *Learn to Play* program. In K. Stagnitti and R. Cooper (eds) *Play as Therapy: Assessment and therapeutic interventions* (pp. 176–86). London: Jessica Kingsley.

Stagnitti, K. (2014). The parent learn to play program: Building relationships through play. In E. Prendiville and J. Howard (eds) *Play Therapy Today: Contemporary practice with individuals, groups and carers* (pp. 149–62). London: Routledge.

Stagnitti, K. (2015). Play, narrative, and children with Autism. In L. Stirling and S. Douglas (eds) *Children's Play, Pretence and Story: Studies in culture, context and ASD*. Melbourne, VIC: Psychological Press.

Stagnitti, K., and Jellie, L. (2006). *Play to Learn: Building literacy in the early years*. Melbourne, VIC: Curriculum Press. Available at: learntoplayevents.com (accessed 30 May 2016).

Stagnitti, K., and Lewis, F.M. (2015). The importance of the quality of preschool children's pretend play ability to the subsequent development of semantic organisation and narrative re-telling skills in early primary school. *International Journal of Speech-Language Pathology*, *17*(2), 148–58.

Stirling, L., Douglas, S., Leekam, S., and Carey, L. (2014). The use of narrative in studying communication in Autism Spectrum Disorders. In J. Arciuli and J. Brock (eds) *Communication in Autism* (pp. 171–215). New York: John Benjamins.

Sunderland, M. (2007). *What Every Parent Needs to Know*. London: Dorling Kindersley.

Whitehead, C., Marchant, J., Craik, D., and Frith, C. (2009). Neural correlates of observing pretend play in which one object is represented as another. *SCAN*, *4*, 369–78.

Whittington, V., and Floyd, I. (2009). Creating intersubjectivity during socio-dramatic play at an Australian kindergarten. *Early Child Development & Care*, *179*, 143–56.

# Discussion and conclusion

*Joan Wilson*

This book has taken us on a journey of consideration of play and expressive arts therapies through the lens of neurobiological development. An introduction to the neurosequential framework was presented, followed by an overview of play therapy approaches that can be appropriately matched to the needs of the client. We then focused our journey on working with the brainstem and midbrain, using the senses to provide calming and a felt sense of safety with clients, to provide reparative experiences of empathic attunement and nurturing presence. We then travelled on through the neurodevelopmental continuum to working with the limbic and cortical systems, promoting emotional regulation and growth, and developing integration of neural networks. In order to plan developmentally appropriate and sequential interventions for clients, whether they are children, adolescents or adults, it is the premise of this book that a working knowledge of neurobiology is necessary. From case conceptualization to intervention planning through to the process of therapy itself, the authors have provided us with clear guidance for our decision-making.

Drawing on a description of Perry's neurosequential model of therapeutics, a framework was presented for conceptualizing developmental stages with matching therapeutic goals and activities. To aid understanding of the stress response system, an overview of Porges' polyvagal theory informed us of the role of the autonomic nervous system to keep us safe in frightening conditions. The survival processes of fight, flight and freeze are regulated by the vagus, a family of nerves originating in the brainstem. Further, the smart (ventral) vagal system, which processes nonverbal cues related to safety and danger (such as facial expressions, voice and movements), describes the connections between the heart and brain that can be utilized to initiate social engagement and implement co-regulation strategies: in other words, to provide a felt sense of safety for the client. Vagal tone is both genetic and experience-dependent, resulting in a wide range of individual differences. Trauma impacts vagal tone, increasing physiological reactivity for the purpose of keeping the individual safe. Neuroception, the sixth sense, develops as a means of assessing the level of risk in the environment. Although this process initially serves the primitive purpose of protection, the result is often hyper- or hypoarousal and an over-appraisal of danger, activating the flight/fight response or immobilization.

Living in a persistent fear state inhibits social engagement and the development of the cortical areas. The smart vagal system, by contrast, supports calming and social engagement when safety is neuroceived, a state that is essential to productive engagement in therapeutic activities. The brain is a social organ, wired for connection, as long as the context is felt to be safe. Our brains rely on other brains to develop, especially under stress. At the most basic level, we look to our caregivers to provide safety and nourishment. When the caregiver is not sensitive and responsive to an infant's needs, neglecting or inflicting trauma on the child, this poses a dilemma, evoking conflicting impulses of attachment-seeking behaviour and pushing away for safety, leaving the child with unmet needs for either safety or nurturance. Early relational trauma at the hands of caregivers sets in place a cascade of post-traumatic effects, developing neural pathways that support defensive and offensive strategies, rather than social connection. The task that lies before the play therapist who is informed by neurosequential development is to identify the areas of the brain affected by the trauma and plan therapeutic interventions to provide reparative experiences, in a bottom–up sequence.

Understanding that neural systems can change, some more easily than others, Perry provides us with the 6 Rs for planning interventions: relational, (developmentally) relevant, repetitive, rewarding, rhythmic and respectful. In order to facilitate state regulation and a sense of safety, the therapist is advised to work neurosequentially, using calming sensory activities at the beginning of therapy, as well as at the beginning of each session. Following that, interventions will be planned to sequentially address the disorganized brain areas. Matching developmental needs with interventions that are respectful of the client's chronological age takes creative planning, with selection from a wide range of play and expressive arts modalities being available.

In the second part of this book, we were invited into the sensory world of the child. The infant is born into a sea of senses, in which they will develop, if conditions are good enough, the ability to experience, process and regulate their senses. The rhythms of breathing, of the heartbeat, of feeding and elimination, and of day and night welcome the child into the world outside the womb. Developing and maintaining homeostasis become the work of the brainstem and midbrain. When insecure attachment or trauma interferes with the development of physiological and emotional regulation, therapeutic interventions involving music and rhythm can support co-regulation, facilitating receptivity to the rhythms and synchronicity of interactions. Attunement and reciprocity, the experience of primary intersubjectivity (the 'we-ness' in relationships), provide a reparative experience for the child who has not yet developed the inner resources to regulate.

Although rhythm and music impact the whole nervous system, the focus here is on the impact on the brainstem and middle brain, which facilitate sensory processing and enable bidirectional communication between the body and the central nervous system. Early attachment experiences, the sense of safety and the ability to communicate are built on sensory and motor capacities of this area of the brain.

The rhythm and music of the infant's world play a fundamental role in achieving homeostasis. In therapy, rhythm and music can play a significant role in creating an environment that fosters these processes, providing opportunities for attunement, mirroring, face-to-face contact and repetition. Shared music and rhythm can access prelinguistic ways of knowing and bring them to the session for healing.

Movement is our first perception *in utero*, with touch embedded in it; these are the foundations on which other senses develop. The first task of the infant after birth is to reconnect with the mother's rhythmic movement, the tone, music and rhythm of her voice, and her unique style of touch. Repetition of this early experience forms implicit memories of the patterns of moving, sensing and responding, providing the context for co-regulation in the attachment relationship. In healthy development, the child learns the world is a safe place, responsive to their needs, and develops the capacity to regulate. When there is developmental trauma, the sequential development of these neuronal patterns is disrupted. With repeated negative experiences, the results of the trauma or neglect become hard-wired into the brain, and the level of homeostasis is altered. The child may constantly perceive threat, even if it is not present, leaving the child either hyperaroused and overreactive or hypoaroused and dissociative. That said, neural systems can change in response to experience. Therapeutic interventions that focus on core regulation (safety, predictability and nurturance) can offer reparative experiences by replicating early, healthy developmental sequences normally experienced in the first 2 years of life. An understanding of the nature and timing of trauma or attachment disruptions assists the therapist in selecting appropriate interventions. Activities involving movement and touch, such as rocking, cradling, dancing and affectionate rough-and-tumble play, offer the child and caregiver opportunities to establish a sense of safety and attunement. Through repetitive experiences of movement and touch, guided by the therapist, the child and caregiver modulate their stress responses and set the stage for further sequential repair.

Sensory experiences are fundamental to homeostasis. Sensory play has the potential to calm or stimulate the nervous system. The sensations are received from the body by the brainstem. Processing and integrating sensory experiences are the work of the midbrain. The five external senses (tactile, olfactory, gustatory, auditory and visual), as well as proprioception (including kinaesthetic awareness, vestibular awareness and visceral awareness), work together to help us sense and organize our perception of our internal and external worlds. Children need to explore and manipulate through sensorimotor play before they can progress to more complex imaginary and symbolic play. Developmental trauma, neglect and hospitalization are examples of ways in which embodiment can be disrupted. Regardless of age, opportunities for sensory and movement play can provide reparative experiences. The outdoor environment is a rich source of sensory experiences. Indoors, a variety of textures, colours, sounds, lighting, smells and tastes can be incorporated into the play room. Tents, cushions, balls, blankets, music, food and aromatic oils are some of the tools that can provide a sensory-rich environment. A range of messy and clean materials allows the client to be drawn to the experience appropriate to them. Implicit memories can often be recalled as a sensory experience, triggered by cues in the present. If the memories are of frightening experiences, attention to the safety of the therapeutic relationship and the safety of the sensory play room is essential to support the client staying in a comfortable state of arousal. A range of approaches to sensory play offer engaging and neurodevelopmentally appropriate interventions that can be offered prescriptively across the age span.

The final part of this book shifted our focus to work with the limbic and cortical areas of the brain – the areas responsible for emotional development and thinking. As we learned in the previous part, attunement originates on a physiological level, experiencing the rhythms of interactions and attending to nonverbal cues (primarily voice, facial expressions and movement). Emotional attunement is a function of the limbic brain, a group of central brain structures that regulates, evaluates and integrates emotional states. When limbic resonance is achieved, each member of the dyad, whether child and caregiver or therapist and client, experiences the sense of being felt by the other; their feeling states resonate, creating the opportunity to co-regulate and experience primary intersubjectivity. An infant's experience of their primary attachment relationship lays down the neural patterns and expectations for future relationships. The therapeutic alliance can reactivate that blueprint in the client, bringing issues to the therapy room for examination and healing.

Whereas senses are the domain of the brainstem and midbrain, images and words are the language of the limbic and cortical areas, with a distinction being made between right and left hemispheric functioning. In overly simplified terms, the right brain is creative and processes emotions, whereas the left brain is more logical and processes thoughts. Right-brain-to-right-brain connection is central to the development of the therapeutic relationship. Identifying which parts of the brain we are working with helps to formulate goals and determine appropriate interventions.

Art therapy uses images as a way of expressing internal realities. As a creative endeavour, art is a right-brained activity, potentially tapping into implicit or non-conscious memories and emotional experiences and engaging the limbic system. When the art has been created, the client is guided to explore the meaning of their work, using words, symbols and metaphors. This begins to cross hemispheres and integrate cortical and limbic functioning (lateral integration). Images also have a powerful effect on our physiological state (vertical integration), increasing the neurological benefits of art therapy. Although the main focus of art therapy is on the higher levels of brain function, all four areas of the brain are involved. State regulation at the brainstem level is foundational, helping the client feel safe in the therapeutic environment. Experimenting with art materials involves the midbrain in the sensory aspect of the experience, allowing the client to embody the experience and move on to higher processes to process difficult emotional material. Connecting body and mind, art therapy supports integration and well-being.

Sandtray therapy is an expressive and projective intervention that gives expression to nonverbalized emotional material. It offers sensory aspects, as well as the safety of therapeutic distance from concerns too difficult to verbalize or bring to the conscious mind. Sandtray therapy does not rely on language and so is suitable for those for whom language is not as well developed. Traumatized clients often demonstrate a delay in speech and language, pointing to the developmental suitability of nonverbal interventions. Furthermore, trauma may involve speechless terror, resulting in traumatized clients being unable to put their intense emotional experience into words. Miniatures become their words, and the sandtray acts as their language of communication. Sandtray therapy also cuts through verbalization or rationalization as a defence, providing a safe means to access deeper material. The embodiment of the sandtray experience allows processing of implicit memory. When the embodied memory is brought into the present and is met with disconfirming experience, the sense of what was missing at the time of the original event, the brain and body are open to new information, providing repair to neural networks. Moving into discussion of the sandtray takes the intervention to the cortical level, integrating the emotional experience with words and making meaning. The importance of the therapeutic relationship providing a safe place to process difficult experiences offers the neurological benefits of physiological state regulation, emotional co-regulation and attachment. In conclusion, sandtray therapy creates opportunities for neurological repair on several levels.

Narrative and storytelling are associated with the limbic and cortical areas of the brain. Imagery and metaphors engage the right hemisphere, whereas the words of the story engage the left. Thus, storytelling supports lateral integration of the hemispheres. The use of play with storytelling further supports right–left hemispheric integration and up–down integration. Developmentally, wordless storytelling precedes verbal storytelling. Storytelling may include play, drama, sand play, art, bibliotherapy, narrative therapy and journaling. Storytelling has played a significant role in history, from legends and myths to family stories to campfire tales. Developing a coherent narrative is correlated with developing more secure forms of attachment. As with other interventions, the creation of a safe place and state regulation is the first step, followed by the development of the therapeutic relationship. The use of storytelling assumes that issues involving lower brain functions have been addressed or are not present prior to beginning the work. In other words, storytelling is prescribed as an intervention within a neurosequential context, addressing higher-level brain functions. The choice of storytelling modalities will depend on the developmental stage of the child, with play and enactment generally being more suitable for younger children, and storytelling, writing or art being more relevant to older clients.

Pretend play, including imaginative play and drama, offers a continuum of complexity to make it applicable across the lifespan. Pretend play emerges in the second year of life and increases in complexity throughout life. Children tell their story, their autobiography, through play. They develop an understanding of the emotional states of others, a theory of mind. Narrative language and self-regulation are woven into the mix. Through pretend play, the child is able to walk into the world of symbolism, representation and social interaction, developing self-representations and their autobiographical narrative. The child learns to read social situations and understand the mental states of others, developing a theory of mind. Beginning with the recognition of self in the mirror and progressing on to role-play and understanding others have different viewpoints, to drama and theatre, the limbic and cortical areas are activated and developed throughout the lifespan. Pretend play offers the opportunity to express various emotions in a safe, contained space and explore scenarios different to those in present life, working towards affect regulation and a sense of mastery. Pretend-play interventions can range from child-centred imaginative play to more complex forms of drama and improvisation, making it suitable for child, adolescent and adult clients. When content becomes too challenging, therapists can introduce activities at a lower brain level to support physiological regulation. As with other therapeutic activities addressing the higher brain levels, pretend play as an intervention is situated on the neurosequential continuum and is selected when earlier-developing areas have been addressed. When children have experienced trauma, therapeutic work is done at the lowest functioning areas of the brain, working up to more complex areas as progress is made, a bottom–up model.

Although the brain is described in segments for the purpose of defining functions and hierarchical development, the neural system is more complex. The various parts of the brain (the central nervous system and the peripheral nervous system) interact through complex networks, integrating functions to synthesize the whole, which is greater than the sum of its parts. Furthermore, as our nervous system is wired to connect, the capacity of one mind to connect with another is as if there is an interpersonal synaptic connection that enables the 'we' to function without losing the 'me'.

Looking at the overall presentation and history of the client, therapists have long been able to make decisions about therapeutic interventions. What has been lacking is an understanding of the neurodevelopmental sequence, which is hierarchical in nature. That is, when an earlier developmental milestone has not been completed, the person does not have the foundation necessary to successfully complete the next. They may develop higher levels of skills, but not be able to access them in times of stress. Incomplete development or damage to specific areas of the brain underlies psychiatric and neurological disorders, as well as some physical ailments. The concepts presented in this book have provided a framework in which to locate the developmental needs of the child and select the matching interventions, targeting areas of earlier brain development and progressing to higher levels when progress is evident. For a client who does not present with a highly aroused stress system, therapeutic interventions can make use of top–down or bottom–up strategies. For clients who have experienced developmental trauma, that is not typically the case. Their nervous systems have an altered set point; they are on the alert for perceived threats; they have developed neural networks to support safety through defensive and offensive strategies, at the expense of the development and use of higher brain functions. This is where we see the top–down approach failing our traumatized clients. Humans need to be in the zone of optimal arousal to be engaged in reparative experiences. Repetitive, rhythmic movement and sensory play can be used as means of targeting the brainstem and midbrain to provide an embodied sense of regulation and safety. Facilitating the felt sense of safety is the first step in creating the crucible in which the therapeutic relationship can develop. When these functions are established, therapeutic work can move on to the limbic and cortical areas. Many of the organizing experiences described in this book target a specific area; that said, the effects may not be limited to that brain function. Lower-level activities may flow into higher-level processing of the experience as the building blocks are set in place. Higher-level interventions may involve sensory experiences to embody and integrate the experience. The nature of many of the modalities allows the sequential progression from one area to another, both over the course of therapy and within sessions. Development of the higher brain functions promotes emotional growth, developing fluidity between body and mind and promoting self-expression, self-awareness and insight. Integration between brain and body functions is developed, which supports flexible and adaptive responses to stress, relationships and overall well-being.

# Index

3Rs of therapy (Bannister) 22, 179
6Rs of therapy (Perry) 27, 171–2, 202

academic stress (case studies) 133–5, 167–8
Achterberg, J. 146
Adlerian play therapy 45–6
adolescents: anorexia case study 75–7; art therapy 149–51; child-centred play therapy 40; development 74–5, 78, 188; drama/imaginative play 65, 188, 193–6; movement/touch therapy 113–14; music/rhythm therapy 94, 95, 97; sandtray therapy 76–7, 132, 133, 165–7; sensory play 130–3; storytelling 179–80
adults (as clients): art therapy 147–9; drama/imaginative play 188–9, 190–1, 196; movement/touch therapy 114–16; music/rhythm therapy 94, 96, 97; sandtray therapy 135, 167–8; sensory play 133–5; storytelling 180–2; Theraplay 44
affect tone 67
'affective neuroscience' 9–10
age-appropriate interventions 27–8
alarm state: as baseline 8–9, 161; normal response to stress 15–16
amygdala 16
Animated Movie Test 194
anorexia nervosa (case study) 75–7
anxiety: music/rhythm therapy 95; sensory play 133–5; on visiting a therapist 29
arousal states 2, 8–9; baseline state 8–9; down- and up-regulation 29, 34, 126; and prolonged stress 16–17, 91; *see also* alarm state; calm state

art therapy 51, 141–55, 204; adolescents 149–51; adults 147–9; affect regulation 145–6; and the media used 60, 61; middle childhood 151–4; trauma-informed expressive arts therapy 61–2; and the unconscious 142–4
attachment 144, 202; musicality and rhythm 84–8; Theraplay 43–4, 128; touch 104, 105; trauma-informed expressive arts therapy 62
autonomic nervous system 2, 15, 88, 89–51, 102–3, 116; polyvagal theory 10–12, 90–1, 103, 201; vagal brake 12, 91
Axline, V. 40

Badenoch, B. 21, 160, 161
Bainbridge Cohen, B. 102
Bannister, A. 22
bidirectionality in regulation 11, 90
bottom–up approach to therapy 2, 9, 143–4, 206; neurological development 8, 88
boundaries 113–14
brain: anatomy 13–14, 89–90; where memories are stored 17–18; *see also* brainstem; cortex
brainstem 2, 24; structure and function 7, 8, 9, 14, 89–90, 126; therapy targeted towards 24, 26–7, 62, 67, 146–7; *see also* movement and touch; music and rhythm; sensory play
breathing regulation 26, 97, 135
Bruner, J. 61

calm state: immobilization without fear 12, 15; restoration after stress response

16; therapy promoting 9, 103; vagal brake 12, 91
carers: conflict between 109–11, 164–7; loss/absence 96, 113–14, 151–4, 177–9, 191–3; role in therapy 34–5, 41–2, 44, 128; *see also* attachment
Carroll, F. 48
Cattanach, A. 48, 49, 65
cerebellum 14, 90
child-centred play therapy (CCPT) 40–1
child clients *see* middle childhood; preschool children
choice bags 131
clinical decision-making 27–8, 65, 202–7
Clyde Findlay, J. 144
cognitive behavioural play therapy (CBPT) 46–7
cognitive behavioural therapy (CBT) 47
cognitive development 123
cognitive impairment in the stress response 16
cognitive/symbolic level of the ETC 61, 62, 71
collective unconscious 42
consonant play 108
co-regulation 11, 105, 203
cortex: and arousal state 9; poorly organised 2; rational brain 13, 14; and theory of mind 191; therapy targeted towards 25, 62, 149, 176–7
cortisol, maternal 86
Cox, M. 144
creative arts therapies 51–2, 59–62; definition 39, 59; *see also* art therapy; drama and imaginative play; movement and touch; music and rhythm
creative level of the ETC 61

Damasio, A. 177
dance therapy 51; *see also* movement and touch
Davies, D. 66
daydreaming 188
defensive systems *see* fight or flight response (hyperarousal); freeze response (hypoarousal)
Developmental Playtherapy 22–3
developmental stage: adolescence 74–5, 78, 188; cognitive development 123; infants 101–2, 105; middle childhood 69–71, 77–8; of play 124, 185–91, 192;
prenatal 102, 104–5; preschool children 24–5, 65–7, 77; and timing of trauma 17–18; *see also* neurosequential model of therapeutics
diencephalon 2, 24, 162
disruptive behaviour in adolescence 165–7
dissociation *see* freeze response (hypoarousal)
documentation of sessions 164
drama and imaginative play 51–2, 64–5, 108, 185–97, 205–6; adolescents 65, 188, 193–6; adults 188–9, 190–1, 196; development 124, 185–91, 192; middle childhood 187–8, 190, 191–3; neurosequential model 189–91; preschool children 186–7

early childhood *see* preschool children
eating disorders (case study) 75–7
echo play 108
egocentric thinking 45, 66
embodied/physical experience of safety 2, 8, 90, 106, 148, 168
Embodiment–Projection–Role (EPR) paradigm 22–3, 124
emotional (mammalian) brain 13, 14; *see also* limbic system
emotional operating systems 9–10, 176
enteric nervous system 103
environment for sensory play 124–5
EPR (Embodiment–Projection–Role) paradigm 22–3, 124
ETC (expressive therapies continuum) model 60–2, 67, 70–1
evidence base 41, 44, 46, 47, 51, 52
explicit memory 13
expressive arts therapies 51–2, 59–62; definition 39, 59; *see also* art therapy; drama and imaginative play; movement and touch; music and rhythm
expressive therapies continuum (ETC) model 60–2, 67, 70–1

false-belief task 190
family members *see* parents
fantasy play *see* drama and imaginative play
Fearn, M. 108–9, 122, 124
fetal environment *see* intrauterine environment

## Index

fight or flight response (hyperarousal) 15–16, 91, 106; down-regulation 29, 126; music therapy in a young child 93–4; in newborns due to *in utero* experiences 86; prolonged 16–17
filial therapy (FT) 41–2
finger-painting 61
freeze response (hypoarousal) 15–16, 91, 106; up-regulation 29, 34, 126
Freud, S. 142

Gaskill, R. 161
gastrointestinal innervation 103
Gestalt play therapy 47–8
Gil, E. 29, 113
Goldschmied, E. 126
Göncü, A. 196
Graves-Alcorn, S.L. 51
Gray, A. 51
Green, E. 51

Hass-Cohen, N. 142
hearing, *in utero* 104
heuristic play 126–7
homeostasis 103, 106, 122, 134, 161; window of tolerance 2, 84, 88–9, 92, 202–3
Homeyer, L. 158, 162
hyperarousal (fight or flight response) 15–16, 91, 106; down-regulation 29, 126; music therapy in a young child 93–4; in newborns due to *in utero* experiences 86; prolonged 16–17
hypoarousal (freeze response) 15–16, 91, 106; up-regulation 29, 34, 126

imaginative play *see* drama and imaginative play
immobilization with fear *see* hypoarousal (freeze response)
immobilization without fear *see* calm state
implicit memory 7–8, 13, 105, 143; preverbal memory 101; sensory memory 121, 125
improvisation 196
infant-directed speech 85, 87
infants: attachment to primary caregiver 84–8, 105; heuristic play 126; needs 27–8, 105; neurodevelopment 101–2, 102–3
interoception 10, 103

intersubjectivity 85–6, 144, 202
intrauterine environment 107; hearing 104; movement and touch 102, 104–5; rhythm 85; stress 86; taste 122

Jennings, S. 22, 107, 124, 185
Jernberg, A. 43
journals, writing 174–5
Jung, C. 142
Jungian play therapy 42–3

Kestly, T. 21, 160
kinesthetic/sensory stage in the ETC 61, 62, 67
Knell, S. 46, 47
Kottman, T. 45
Kuhn-Popp, N. 190

Landgarten, H. 60
language: infant-directed speech 85, 87; providing a means of expression 35
Learn to Play therapy 191–6
Lee, A. 50
left hemisphere of the brain 13, 144–5, 177
limbic system 9–10, 14, 176, 204; implicit memory 13; limbic resonance between therapist and client 144–5; stress response 16; therapy targeted towards 24–5, 62; *see also* art therapy; sandtray therapy; storytelling
loss/absence of parents/carers (case studies) 96, 113–14, 151–4, 164–5, 177–9, 191–3
loss of a partner (case study) 196
Lowenfeld, M. 158

McNiff, S. 154
magical thinking 66, 70
make-believe play *see* drama and imaginative play
Malchiodi, C. 39, 51, 62
malleable materials 95
mammalian (emotional) brain 13, 14; *see also* limbic system
media used in art therapy 60, 61
medical trauma in young children 67–9
memory 17–18; explicit (left-brain) 13; implicit (right-brain) 7–8, 13, 101–2, 105, 143; sensory 121, 125
messy play 28, 95, 127–8, 131

metaphor use in therapy 145, 173
midbrain 7, 9, 14, 90
middle childhood 69–73, 77–8; art therapy 151–4; drama/imaginative play 187–8, 190, 191–3; movement and touch in therapy 111–13; sandtray therapy 72–3, 164–5; sensory play 128–30
Mills, J. 49
mimicry 108
miniatures, in sandtray therapy 72–3, 76, 159, 162, 164–8
mirror neurons 108
mirroring 92–3, 94, 108–9
modes of representation (Bruner) 61
monster masks 64
moral development 70
motherese (infant-directed speech) 85, 87
mother–infant bond 84–8, 105
motivational circuits 9–10, 176
movement and touch 101–17, 203; adolescents 113–14; adults 114–16; in early development 101–2, 104–5; middle childhood 111–13; preschool children 109–11; sensory play 124; skin is the organ of touch 103–4, 122; therapist's self-awareness 109
Munns, E. 43
music and rhythm 51, 83–98, 108, 202–3; adolescents 94, 95, 97; adults 94, 96, 97; attachment with the primary caregiver 84–8; making music 97; as part of sensory play 133, 134; preschool children 93–4; preterm babies 86

naming of drawn objects 63
naming emotions in storytelling 176
Naparstek, B. 148
narrative play therapy 48–9, 174; *see also* storytelling
neglect: case studies 96, 111–13, 128–30, 179–80; definition 105–6
neocortex: and arousal state 9; rational brain 13, 14; and theory of mind 191; therapy targeted towards 25, 62, 149, 176–7; underdeveloped 2
neuroception 10–11, 91, 201–2
neurosequential model of therapeutics 8–9, 23–34, 88–92, 201–2, 206–7;

adolescence 74–7, 78; and art therapy 146–7; and the ETC model 61–2; memory 17–18; middle childhood 69–73, 77–8; preschool children 24–5, 65–9, 77; and pretend play 189–91; and sandtray therapy 161–2; and sensory play 125–6, 134; and storytelling 175–7; and various types of play therapy 42, 44, 48, 49, 50, 52
newborn infants 85–7, 102, 105
nonverbal cues 12, 35

Oaklander, V. 47
outdoor play 124

Pally, R. 145
panic attacks 133–5, 147–9
Panksepp, J. 9, 90
parasympathetic nervous system *see* vagal system
parents: conflict between 109–11, 164–7; loss/absence 96, 113–14, 151–4, 177–9, 191–3; role in therapy 34–5, 41–2, 44, 128; *see also* attachment
passing games 94
Pate, J. 168
Pennebaker, J.W. 174
perceptual/affective level of the ETC 61, 62, 70
peripheral nervous system (PNS) 15
Perone, A. 196
Perry, B.D. 8–9, 18, 23, 26, 27, 102, 105–6, 160, 161, 162, 168, 177, 189
physical contact between client and therapist 94
physical play 22–3, 124
Piaget, J. 123
play-dough 95, 178
play therapy: age-appropriate 27–8; definition 39; developmental play therapy 22–3, 107–9; directive approach 43–4; non-directive approach 40–3; variable approach 45–50; why it works 10, 105–6; *see also* drama and imaginative play; sensory play
play therapy dimensions model 63
polyvagal theory 10–12, 90–1, 103, 201
Porges, S.W. 10–12, 35, 90–1, 103
prenatal environment *see* intrauterine environment

preschool children 24–5, 65–9, 77; drama/imaginative play 186–7; movement and touch in therapy 109–11; music/rhythm therapy 93–4; sensory play 126–7; storytelling 177–9
pretend play (drama and imaginative play) 51–2, 64–5, 108, 185–97, 205–6; adolescents 65, 188, 193–6; adults 188–9, 190–1, 196; development 124, 185–91, 192; middle childhood 187–8, 190, 191–3; preschool children 186–7
proprioception 121–2
protoconversations 85, 87
psychodynamic play therapy 49–50
puppets 66
putty 95

questioning skills 63–4

rational brain 13, 14; *see also* cortex
reassurance 22, 146, 179
re-enactment 22, 179
rehearsal 22, 179
repatterning 106; in case study 111
representational play *see* drama and imaginative play
reptilian brain 13, 14
research results 41, 44, 46, 47, 51, 52
rhythm *see* music and rhythm
right hemisphere of the brain 89; memory 7–8, 13, 101–2, 109, 143; right-brain-to-right-brain communication 144–5, 204; sandtray therapy 161; storytelling 177; Theraplay 44
risk evaluation 10–11, 91
rule-based play 112
Ryan, V. 40

safety (in therapy) 8, 11, 22, 29, 204; art therapy 143, 146; narrative therapy 174; sandtray therapy 162
sand play therapy 158
sandtray therapy 157–69, 205; adolescents 76–7, 132, 133, 165–7; adults 135, 167–8; benefits 158–60; methods 162–4; middle childhood 72–3, 164–5; and neurobiology 160–2
Schaverien, J. 144
Schögler, B. 92
Schore, A. 101–2, 104, 144–5

selective mutism (case study) 130–3
self-harm (case study) 149–51; *see also* eating disorders (case study)
self-representation 186, 190
sensory boxes 131
sensory memory 121, 125
sensory play 121–35, 203–4; adolescents 130–3; adults 133–5; external and internal senses 121–2; infants 126; kinesthetic/sensory stage in the ETC 61, 62, 67; middle childhood 128–30; preschool children 126–7
sexual abuse/assault: on an adult 114–16, 180–2; on a child 111–13
Shore, R. 175
Siegal, D. 161
skills and techniques used by psychotherapists 59–78
skin 103–4, 122
smell, sense of 122
social behaviour in adolescents 74–5, 188, 193–6
social constructionism 174
social engagement, and the vagal system 11–12, 91, 103
somatic nervous system 15
Stagnitti, K. 191
StoryPlay 49
storytelling 64–5, 171–82, 205; adolescents 179–80; adults 180–2; narrative play therapy 48–9, 174; preschool children 177–9
stress: effect of prolonged stress on arousal state 16–17, 91; normal stress response 15–16; prenatal/neonatal 86, 91
Sunderland, M. 13
Sweeney, D. 157–8, 158, 162
symbolic play 65, 76, 130, 173
sympathetic nervous system 15, 91

talking therapy 7, 47
taste, sense of 122
theory of mind 186–7, 189, 190–1
therapeutic distance in sandtray therapy 159
therapeutic relationship 10, 106–7, 144; *see also* safety (in therapy)
therapeutic touchstone 112, 130
Theraplay 43–4, 128
Thielgaard, A. 144

top–down approach to therapy 2, 143–4
touch *see* movement and touch
transference: in art therapy 142; in sandtray therapy 159
trauma: in an adult 147–9; in a child 67–9; definition 105; memory of 7–8, 13, 17; neurological patterns 105; play therapy 10, 68–9; sandtray therapy 159, 160–2; timing 17–18
trauma-informed expressive arts therapy 61–2
treasure baskets 126
Trevarthen, C. 84, 85, 87, 90, 92
triune brain 13–14

unconscious mind: and art therapy 142–4; collective unconscious 42

vagal system 2, 15, 103; polyvagal theory 10–12, 90–1, 103, 201; vagal brake 12, 91
Vance, R. 143
van der Kolk, B.A. 23, 168
vestibulocochlear nerve 104

Wahlin, K. 143
Weinrib, E. 164
Whitehead, C. 190
Wilkinson, M. 143
Wilson, K. 40
'window of tolerance' (homeostasis) 2, 84, 88–9, 92, 202–3
writing as therapy 174–5

young children *see* preschool children